PERMISSION TO *FEEL*

PERMISSION TO

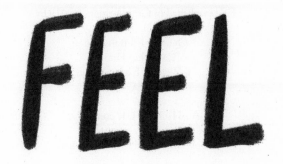

FEEL

UNLOCK THE POWER OF EMOTIONS TO HELP YOURSELF AND YOUR CHILD THRIVE

Professor Marc Brackett

Quercus

First published in the US in 2019 by Celadon Books,
a division of Macmillan Publishers

First published in Great Britain in 2019 by

Quercus Editions Ltd
Carmelite House
50 Victoria Embankment
London EC4Y 0DZ

An Hachette UK company

A CIP catalogue record for this book is available from the British Library

TPB ISBN 978 1 78747 881 7
Ebook ISBN 978 1 78747 883 1

10 9 8 7 6 5 4 3 2 1

Typeset by Jouve (UK), Milton Keynes

Printed and bound in Great Britain by Clays Ltd, Elcograf S.p.A.

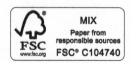

Papers used by Quercus Editions Ltd are from well-managed
forests and other responsible sources.

For Uncle Marvin
And Mom and Dad

Contents

PART THREE: APPLYING EMOTION SKILLS FOR OPTIMUM
WELL-BEING AND SUCCESS

Prologue

OKAY, LET'S GET THE easy questions out of the way first: What's up with that title? Since when does anybody need permission to feel?

True, we all have feelings more or less continuously, every waking moment—even in our dreams—without ever asking or getting anybody's approval. To stop feeling would be like to stop thinking. Or breathing. Impossible. Our emotions are a big part—maybe the biggest part—of what makes us human.

And yet we go through life trying hard to pretend otherwise. Our true feelings can be messy, inconvenient, confusing, even addictive. They leave us vulnerable, exposed, naked to the world. They make us do things we wish we hadn't done. It's no wonder our emotions scare us sometimes—they seem so out of our control. Too often we do our best to deny them or hide them—even from ourselves. Our attitudes about them get passed along to our children, who learn by taking their cues from us, their parents and teachers—their role models. Our kids receive the message loud and clear, so that before long, they, too, have learned to suppress even the most urgent messages from deep inside their beings. Just as we learned to do.

You haven't even begun reading this book yet, but I'll bet you already know what I'm talking about.

So, we deny ourselves—and one another—the permission to feel. We suck it up, squash it down, act out. We avoid the difficult conversation with our colleague; we explode at a loved one; and we helplessly go through an entire bag of cookies and have no idea why. When we deny ourselves the permission to feel, a long list of unwanted outcomes ensues. We lose the ability to even identify what we're feeling—it's like, without noticing, we go a little numb inside. When that happens, we're unable to understand why we're experiencing an emotion or what's happening in our lives that's causing it. Because of that we're unable to name it, so we can't express it, either, in terms the people around us would understand. And when we can't recognize, understand, or put into words what we feel, it's impossible for us to do anything about it: to master our feelings—not to deny them but to accept them all, even embrace them—and learn to make our emotions work for us, not against us.

I spend every minute of my working life dealing with these issues. Through academic research and plenty of real-life experience, especially in the world of education, I've seen the terrible cost of our inability to deal in healthy ways with our emotional lives.

Here's some evidence:

- In 2017, about 8 percent of adolescents aged twelve to seventeen and 25 percent of young adults aged eighteen to twenty-five were current users of illicit drugs.
- The number of incidents of bullying and harassment in U.S. K–12 schools reported to the Anti-Defamation League doubled each year between 2015 and 2017.
- According to a 2014 Gallup poll, 46 percent of teachers report high daily stress during the school year. That's tied with nurses for the highest rate among all occupational groups.

- A 2018 Gallup poll revealed that over 50 percent of employees are unengaged at work; 13 percent of those are "miserable."
- From 2016–2017, more than one in three students across 196 U.S. college campuses reported diagnosed mental health conditions. Some campuses have reported a 30 percent increase in mental health problems per year.
- According to the 2019 World Happiness Report, negative feelings, including worry, sadness, and anger, have been rising around the world, up by 27 percent from 2010 to 2018.
- Anxiety disorders are the most common mental illness in the U.S., affecting 25 percent of children between thirteen and eighteen years old.
- Depression is the leading cause of disability worldwide.
- Worldwide mental health problems could cost the global economy up to $16 trillion by 2030. These include direct costs of health care and medicines or other therapies and indirect costs such as loss of productivity.

We seem to prefer spending more money and effort on dealing with the results of our emotional problems rather than trying to prevent them.

I have a personal interest in the bad things that happen when we deny ourselves permission to feel. Meaning I've been there, but thanks to someone who cared, I made it out alive. We'll talk about that too.

Only a few naturally insightful among us can claim to have the skills discussed in this book without consciously pursuing them. I had to learn them. And these *are* skills. All personality types—loud or quiet, imaginative or practical, neurotic or happy-go-lucky—will find them accessible and even life-changing. These are clear, simple, and tested skills that can be acquired by anyone of almost any age.

Recently, I was training administrators in one of the country's most challenging school districts. I was warned, "They'll eat you alive." At lunch on the first day, I was standing in the buffet line next to a principal, and to make small talk, I asked him, "So, what do you think about the session so far?" He looked me in the eye, then looked down at the food and said, "The desserts look pretty good." I realized at that moment what I was up against. I'm used to resistance, but his attitude hit hard. I decided at that moment that he was going to be my project. His superintendent was fully on board, but it was clear that we would succeed in this district only if principals, like this guy, were also believers.

At the end of a couple of days of intensive teaching, I ran into him again. "The other day, when we met, you weren't so sure this course was going to work for you," I said. "I'm curious. Now that you've spent two days learning about emotions and how to integrate emotion skills into your school, what do you think?"

"Well, I'll tell you," he said, pausing to collect his thoughts. "I realize now that I didn't know what I didn't know. The language of feelings was foreign to me."

That was encouraging, I thought. Then he went on.

"So, thank you for giving me the permission to feel."

Let's begin there.

PART ONE

PERMISSION TO FEEL

1

Permission to Feel

How are you feeling?

Given the subject of this book, it's a reasonable question. I may ask it more than once before we're through. In theory, given that it's something we're asked so often in one form or another, that should make it the easiest question ever, instead of the hardest—depending on how honest we're going to be when we answer.

I'm speaking now not only as a psychologist and director of a center devoted to emotional well-being but also as a fellow human. To be perfectly honest, I wish someone had asked me that question when I was a kid—asked it and really, truly, wanted to know the answer and had the courage to do something about what I would have revealed.

I was not a happy child.

I felt scared, angry, hopeless. Bullied. Isolated. And I suffered.

Boy, did I suffer.

When I was in middle school, you only had to look at me to see that something was seriously wrong. I was a poor student in school, mostly

Cs and Ds. My eating was so messed up that I went from severely thin to overweight. I had no real friends.

My parents loved me and cared for me—I knew that. But they had their own miseries. Mom was anxious and depressed and had a drinking problem. Dad was raging, scary, and disappointed in a son who wasn't as tough as he was. But they had at least one thing in common: no clue about how to deal with feelings—neither their own nor mine.

I would spend hours alone in my room, crying or anguishing over the bullying I silently endured at school. But my main response to life was rage. I would talk back to my mother, yell, scream. "Who do you think you are to talk to me like that?" she would holler back. "Wait till your father gets home!" When he did, my mother would tell him how I had mistreated her, and then he would storm into my room, shouting, "If I have to tell you one more time to stop speaking to your mother that way, I'm going to lose it!" Sometimes he'd spare me the lecture and just start hitting.

Then my mother would jump in, and the two of them would battle over how he was handling the situation. Finally, he would give up, and my mother would come into my room and say, "Marc, I saved you *this* time . . ."

I wondered: What did she think she had saved me from?

Without meaning to, they taught me a powerful lesson. Keep my feelings to myself. Definitely do not allow my parents to see them. That would just make a bad scene worse.

This was around the time they learned my most terrible secret—that a neighbor, a friend of the family, had been sexually abusing me. When my parents finally found out, my father grabbed a bat from the basement and nearly killed the man. My mother almost had a nervous breakdown. The police came and arrested the neighbor, and soon the whole neighborhood knew. It turned out my abuser had been violating dozens of other children as well.

You'd think everyone would be glad that I had come forward and exposed this horror. But you'd be wrong. I became an instant pariah.

Every adult warned their kids to stay away from me. The bullying got even worse.

Suddenly, the source of my constant emotional meltdowns was clear to my parents. My bad grades. My bulimia. My social isolation. My despair. My rage.

My parents did what many people do under similar pressures.

They freaked out.

That's not entirely accurate—they knew enough to send me to a therapist. They were too overwhelmed by their own problems, just trying to survive, to be able to deal with anybody else's emotional life. They either missed or ignored all the signals I was sending, which doesn't really come as a surprise. Maybe they felt safer not asking too many questions about my life at school or in our neighborhood. Maybe they were afraid of what they'd find out—afraid that once they knew, they'd have to do something about it.

Perhaps if their parents had asked them the right questions, and taught them how to deal with their feelings and what to do when problems arose, my life back then might have been different. Maybe my parents would have been able to see the pain I was in and know how to help me.

Never happened.

Some of this may sound familiar to you. In my line of work, I meet a lot of people who spent their childhoods as I did. Unseen, unacknowledged, bad feelings buried deep inside. No two stories are identical. People tell me how they were physically abused. Or ignored and silenced. Or made to suffer emotional abuse. Or smothered by parents who lived vicariously through them. Or neglected by parents who were alcoholics or addicts. It's our responses that are the same.

Sometimes the tales aren't nearly so dramatic—just people who grew up in homes where everyday emotional issues were ignored because no one had ever learned how to talk about them or take actions to address them. Your life didn't have to be tragic for you to feel as though your emotional life didn't matter to anyone but you.

Here's how I responded: I became numb to how I felt. I was under emotional lockdown. Survival mode.

And then a miracle took place.

Its name was Marvin. Uncle Marvin, actually.

He was my mother's brother, a schoolteacher by day and a bandleader at night and on the weekends. Our family would travel from New Jersey up to the resorts in the Catskill Mountains to see our family celebrity perform. Uncle Marvin was truly an outlier—unique among all my relatives and every other adult I knew. He was like the Robin Williams character in *Dead Poets Society*.

In his day job, even back then in the 1970s, Uncle Marvin was trying to create a curriculum that would encourage students to express how they felt. He believed it was the missing link in their education—that *emotion skills* would improve their learning and their lives. I would help Uncle Marvin by typing his notes as he read them aloud. I encountered terms such as "despair," "alienation," "commitment," and "elation" and recognized myself in many of them.

One summer afternoon, while we were sitting in our backyard together, he asked if he could give me an IQ test. Turns out that I was smarter than my dismal report cards suggested. I also think he suspected that I had a lot of turmoil going on deep inside having to do with school and being abused. It led Uncle Marvin to ask me a question I had rarely, if ever, heard coming from an adult or anyone else:

"Marc," he said, "how are you feeling?"

With those words, the dam inside me broke, and out came the torrent. Every horrible thing I was experiencing at the time, and every feeling I had in response, all came tumbling out in a rush.

That one little question was all it took to change my life. It wasn't just what he said, it was the way he said it. Truly wanting to hear the answer. Not judging me for what I felt. He just listened, openly and with empathy, to what I was expressing. He didn't try to interpret me or explain me.

I really let loose that day.

"I have no real friends, I suck at sports, I'm fat, and the kids at school all hate me," I wailed, sobbing.

Uncle Marvin just listened. He heard me out. My uncle was the first person who had ever chosen not to focus on my outward behavior—snarky, withdrawn, defiant, definitely unpleasant to be around—and instead sensed that something else was going on, something significant that no one, not even I, had acknowledged.

Uncle Marvin gave me permission to feel.

Given all that, it's no surprise that for the past twenty-five years I've been researching and writing about emotions and running around the world talking to people about their feelings. It's become my passion and my life's work. I'm a professor in the Yale Child Study Center and founding director of the Yale Center for Emotional Intelligence. At the center, I lead a team of scientists and practitioners who conduct research on emotions and emotion skills and develop approaches to teach people of all ages—from preschoolers to CEOs—the skills that can help them thrive. Our center's goal is to use the power of emotions to create a healthier and more equitable, innovative, and compassionate society.

Each year I give dozens of talks to educators, schoolchildren, parents, business executives, entrepreneurs, political leaders, scientists, medical practitioners, and every other kind of person you can imagine, all over the world. My message for everyone is the same: that if we can learn to identify, express, and harness our feelings, even the most challenging ones, we can use those emotions to help us create positive, satisfying lives.

Whenever I speak to a group, I start by asking people to spend a few minutes thinking about how they're feeling right in the moment. Then I call on them to share. Their answers reveal a lot—not necessarily about their emotions but about our difficulty in discussing our emotional lives. What I find is that we don't even have the vocabulary to describe our feelings in useful detail—three-quarters of the people have a hard time coming up with a "feeling" word. When the words do come, they don't usually tell us very much. People fumble around a bit, hem and haw, and then use the most commonplace terms we all rely on—*I feel fine, good, okay . . .*

It makes you wonder: Do I even know how I'm feeling? Have I given myself permission to ask? Have I ever really asked my partner, my child, my colleague? Today, when nearly every question can be handled instantly by Siri, or Google, or Alexa, we're losing the habit of pausing to look inward, or to one another, for answers. But even Siri doesn't know everything. And Google can't tell you why your son or daughter is feeling hopeless or excited, or why your significant other feels not so significant lately, or why you can't shake that chronic low-level anxiety that plagues you.

It makes perfect sense that we're uncomfortable and awkward when expressing our emotional lives. This is true even when we're experiencing positive feelings. But it's especially so when they're unpleasant—sad, resentful, scared, rejected. Those all connect us to our weaknesses, and who wants to show those off? The instinct to protect ourselves by hiding our vulnerability is natural. Even animals in the wild do it. It's self-preservation, pure and simple.

And yet we all ask this question or something like it countless times a day, and we're called on to answer it just as often:

How are you? How are you doing? How are you feeling?

We ask it so reflexively that we scarcely hear ourselves. And we answer in the same spirit:

Great, thanks, how are you? Everything's fine! Busy!

Without pausing for even a second to think before we reply.

It's one of the great paradoxes of the human condition—we ask some variation of the question "How are you feeling?" over and over, which would lead one to assume that we attach some importance to it. And yet we never expect or desire—or provide—an honest answer.

Imagine what would happen if next time an acquaintance (or the barista at Starbucks) says, "Hi, how are you?" you were to stop and take the next five minutes to give a detailed—unedited—response. Really bare your soul. I guarantee it would be a long time before that particular person inquired again.

There's something meaningful going on in there—in that huge disconnect between our willingness to ask how we feel and our reluctance to respond thoughtfully. We now know that, aside maybe from physical health, our emotional state is one of the most important aspects of our lives. It rules everything else. Its influence is pervasive. Yet it is also the thing we steer around most carefully. Our inner lives are uncharted territory even to us, a risky place to explore.

Our lives are saturated with emotions—sadness, disappointment, anxiety, irritation, enthusiasm, and even tranquility. Sometimes— often—those feelings are inconvenient. They get in the way of our busy lives, or at least that's what we tell ourselves. So we do our best to ignore them. It's everywhere, from the stiff upper lip of our country's Puritan founders to the tough-it-out ethos of schoolyards and playgrounds. We all believe that our feelings are important and deserve to be addressed respectfully and fully. But we also think of emotions as being disruptive and unproductive—at work, at home, and everywhere else. Until the 1980s, most psychologists viewed emotions as extraneous noise, useless static. Our feelings slow us down and get in the way of achieving our goals. We've all heard the message: Get over it. Stop focusing on yourself (as though such a thing were possible!). Don't be so sensitive. Time to move on.

The irony, though, is that when we ignore our feelings, or suppress them, they only become stronger. The really powerful emotions build up inside us, like a dark force that inevitably poisons everything we do, whether we like it or not. Hurt feelings don't vanish on their own. They don't heal themselves. If we don't express our emotions, they pile up like a debt that will eventually come due.

And I'm not talking only about the times we're feeling something unpleasant. We may also fail to understand exactly how we feel when things are going great. We're content just to enjoy the emotions and not probe too deeply. It's a mistake, of course. If we're going to make positive choices in the future, we need to know what will bring us happiness—and why.

Proof of our inability to deal constructively with our emotional lives is all around us. In 2015, in collaboration with the Robert Wood Johnson Foundation and Born This Way Foundation (founded by Lady Gaga and her mother, Cynthia Germanotta), we conducted a large-scale survey of twenty-two thousand teenagers from across the United States and asked them to describe how they feel while in school. Three-quarters of the words they used were negative, with "tired," "bored," and "stressed" topping the list. This wasn't surprising given that around 30 percent of elementary and middle school students now experience adjustment problems severe enough to require regular counseling. In economically disadvantaged schools, this runs as high as 60 percent.

American youths now rank in the bottom quarter among developed nations in well-being and life satisfaction, according to a report by UNICEF. Research shows that our youths have stress levels that surpass those of adults. Our teenagers are now world leaders in violence, binge drinking, marijuana use, and obesity. More than half of college students experience overwhelming anxiety, and a third report intense depression. And over the last two decades, there has been a 28 percent increase in our suicide rate.

How clearly will kids think when they are feeling tired, bored, and stressed? How well do they absorb new information when they are anxious? Do they take their studies seriously? Do they feel inclined to express their curiosity and pursue learning?

Here's a story that tells me a lot about the emotional atmosphere in schools.

The superintendent of a major metropolitan district was out making classroom visits. As she walked the halls with the principal, she saw a little girl headed to a classroom and greeted her, attempting to start up a conversation.

The girl refused to acknowledge her.

"She wouldn't say hello to me," the superintendent told me. After a moment of mutual confusion, the little girl put her head down and continued on her way. Apparently, students had been told they could walk only on the white line painted down the middle of the corridors. "Stepping over to talk to me would mean breaking the rules," said the superintendent.

We'll never know how that conversation might have gone. The natural instinct of both student and educator to engage with each other was squelched by the school's demand for order above all else.

What can happen in a single exchange? A moment of small talk in a hallway? Probably very little. Although if you are like me, you have some memories from early childhood that stand out from the fog of years, that have endured over time for no other reason than that a grown-up made space in his or her life, for a moment, for you. A small thing like that, if it is heartfelt, can reverberate.

It's not only students who feel oppressed. What about their teachers? In 2017, in collaboration with the New Teacher Center, we surveyed more than five thousand educators and found that they spend nearly 70 percent of their workdays feeling "frustrated," "overwhelmed," and "stressed." This conforms with Gallup data showing that nearly half of U.S. teachers report high stress on a daily basis. A frightening snapshot of our educational system, wouldn't you agree?

How effective are our educators when they feel just as frustrated, overwhelmed, and stressed as the kids? Will they give 100 percent to their lessons? Do they snap at students unintentionally, or ignore their needs, because they are emotionally exhausted? Are they leaving work feeling burned out, dreading tomorrow's return to the classroom?

If we don't understand emotions and find strategies to deal with them, they will take over our lives, as they did for me as a child. Fear and anxiety made it impossible for me to try to deal with my problems. I was paralyzed. The science now proves why. If there had been someone to teach me the skills—if there had been someone to even tell me there *were* such skills—I might have felt more in control of my situation. Instead, all I could do was endure it.

During presentations, I'll often make the observation that many children today are in serious crisis mode. Usually this will prompt someone to ask a question that's really more of an opinion: "Don't you think these kids lack the toughness and moral fiber that people had generations ago?"

My response to this has matured over the years. Once, a statement like that would really rile me. It sounded like somebody looking for a reason to feel superior and blame the victims. Now I think it's irresponsible.

Let's suppose that children today *do* lack the emotional strength we, or some other generation, had in abundance. Let's assume that in the past kids were just as challenged—maybe more—but they were able to buckle down and deal with it.

So what?

Would that mean we abdicate responsibility for doing our best to help today's kids? If they do require a little help, isn't it our job to give it to them, without judging? And if they need so much support, how did they end up that way? Did it have anything to do with how we raised them?

There was a time, not so long ago, that children did have a serious need that was not being met. Our national response was instructive. In 1945, while World War II was still raging, a general (and former teacher) named Lewis B. Hershey testified before Congress that almost half of all army draftees were turned away for reasons owing to poor nutrition. He was in a good position to know: Hershey was in charge of the Selective Service System. He saw the underfed and malnourished young American men and realized their unfitness for war.

Congress did not issue a proclamation condemning the fecklessness of the younger generation. It passed a bipartisan bill: the National School Lunch Act.

In other words, we fed our kids.

. . .

It's time to feed our kids again.

At the Yale Center for Emotional Intelligence, that's all we think about: how we can help people to identify their emotions, understand the influence of their feelings on all aspects of their lives, and develop the skills to make sure they use their emotions in healthy, productive ways.

Once, after a talk to mental health professionals at a major hospital, the head of child psychiatry approached me. He said, "Marc, great job. But, you know, according to our data we're going to need another eight thousand child psychiatrists to deal with the problems these kids will be having."

I was stunned.

"You misunderstood me. I want to put you all out of business," I said half-jokingly.

He was thinking that all those troubled children would need professional interventions in order to deal with their lives. I was saying that we need to remake education so that it includes emotion skills—so that professional interventions become less necessary.

It's been nearly thirty years since the idea of emotional intelligence was introduced by my mentors, Peter Salovey, professor of psychology and current president of Yale University, and Jack Mayer, professor of psychology at the University of New Hampshire. It's been a quarter century since Daniel Goleman published his bestselling book *Emotional Intelligence*, which popularized the concept. And yet we're still grappling with the most basic questions, such as "How are you feeling?"

Feelings are a form of information. They're like news reports from inside our psyches, sending messages about what's going on inside the unique person that is each of us in response to whatever internal or external events we're experiencing. We need to access that information and then figure out what it's telling us. That way we can make the most informed decisions.

That's a major challenge. It's not as though every emotion comes with a label telling us precisely what prompted it, and why, and what can be done to resolve it. Our thinking and behavior absolutely change in response to what we're feeling. But we don't always know why or how best to address our emotions. For parents, this might be a familiar scenario: we see a child who's clearly suffering, and the reason isn't apparent. Ask simply, "What's wrong?" and the answer will almost never reveal the source of the anguish. Maybe the child doesn't even know what's wrong.

Here's an example: Anger can sometimes seem unprovoked or inexplicable, but in almost every case it's a response to what we perceive as unfair treatment. We've suffered an injustice of some kind, big or small, and it makes us mad. Someone cut in front of you in line—and you're irritated. You were up for a promotion at work, but it went to the boss's niece—and you're outraged. But it's the same basic dynamic at work.

Most of us don't enjoy dealing with anger, whether it's our own or someone else's. When a parent or teacher is faced with what might appear to be an angry child, often the first impulse is to threaten discipline—if you don't stop yelling, or speaking rudely, or stamping your feet, you'll go sit in the corner, or I'll send you to your room, or you'll lose your privileges!

When it's an adult who's angry, our response isn't much different. We immediately pull back. We stop listening sympathetically. We feel under attack, which makes it nearly impossible for us to deal with the information the person is conveying. But that anger was an important message. If we can try to mollify the injustice that sparked it, the anger will go away, because it's outlived its usefulness. If not, it will fester, even if it seems to subside.

Thankfully, there's a science to understanding emotion. It's not just a matter of intuition, opinion, or gut instinct. We are not born with an innate talent for recognizing what we or anyone else is feeling and why. We all have to learn it. *I* had to learn it.

As with any science, there's a process of discovery, a method of investigation. After three decades of research and practical experience, we at the Yale Center have identified the talents needed to become what we've termed an "emotion scientist."

Here are the five skills we've identified. We need to

- recognize our own emotions and those of others, not just in the things we think, feel, and say but in facial expressions, body language, vocal tones, and other nonverbal signals.
- understand those feelings and determine their source—what experiences actually caused them—and then see how they've influenced our behaviors.
- label emotions with a nuanced vocabulary.
- express our feelings in accordance with cultural norms and social contexts in a way that tries to inform and invites empathy from the listener.
- regulate emotions, rather than let them regulate us, by finding practical strategies for dealing with what we and others feel.

The rest of this book is devoted to teaching those skills and how to use them.

In the late 1990s, Uncle Marvin and I set out together to bring these skills to schools. We failed. We were prepared to deliver classroom instruction only to children. But some teachers were resistant. "Teaching kids about anxiety makes me nervous," one said. "I'm not opening that Pandora's box of talking about how these kids feel," said another. If the teachers didn't believe in the importance of these emotion skills, they'd never be effective at instructing their students. So Marvin and I, along with new colleagues at Yale, went back to the drawing board. We saw that we would never reach children until we first enlisted teachers who understood the importance of emotion skills. And soon after that we realized that only if there was commitment at the very top, at the school board, superintendent, and principal levels, could entire school systems be transformed.

Then it became clear that the skills must be even more widely shared. We adults *all* need to understand how our emotions influence us and everyone around us, not just schoolchildren. We need to develop the skills and be positive role models. Educators and parents have to demonstrate the ability to identify, discuss, and regulate their own emotions before they can teach the skills to others. Our classroom research shows that where there is an emotionally skilled teacher present, students disrupt less, focus more, and perform better academically. Our studies show that where there is an emotionally skilled principal, there are teachers who are less stressed and more satisfied. And where there is an emotionally skilled parent, there are children who have a greater ability to identify and regulate their emotions.

Once our children grow into emotionally skilled adults, the entire culture will change—for the better. But learning the skills and improving the way we respond to our feelings doesn't mean we'll suddenly become happy all the time. Perpetual happiness can't be our goal—it's just not how real life works. We need the ability to experience and express all emotions, to down- or up-regulate both pleasant and unpleasant emotions in order to achieve greater well-being, make the most informed decisions, build and maintain meaningful relationships, and realize our potential.

But that starts with all of us. If you're a parent, ask yourself this: What are the qualities you most want your children to possess as they grow into adults? Is it math skills, scientific knowledge, athletic ability? Or is it confidence, kindness, a sense of purpose, the wisdom to build healthy, lasting relationships? When we consult with corporations, they tell us they're searching for employees who persevere with a task, who take personal responsibility for their work, who can get along with others and function as members of a team. Not technical abilities or specialized knowledge—they're looking first for emotional attributes. A colleague from the RAND Corporation told me that technology advances so rapidly today that companies don't hire workers for their current skills—firms are looking for people who are flexible, who can present new ideas, inspire cooperation in groups, manage and lead teams, and so on.

We may acquire some of those skills by osmosis—by watching and emulating others who possess them. But for the most part they must be taught. And they are best learned in communities. Emotion skills are both personal and mutual. They can be used privately, but their best application is throughout a community, so that a network emerges to reinforce its own influence. I have seen this happen—these skills are being deployed in thousands of schools all over the world, with dramatic results. The children benefit, naturally: there is less bullying and emotional distress, better attendance, fewer suspensions, and greater academic achievement. But we have also seen that schools where these skills are taught have teachers with lower levels of stress and burnout, fewer intentions to leave the profession, greater job satisfaction, and more engaging classrooms.

We all want our lives, and the lives of the people we love, to be free of hardship and troubling events.

We can never make that happen.

We all want our lives to be filled with healthy relationships, compassion, and a sense of purpose.

That we can make happen.

Uncle Marvin showed me how. It starts with the permission to feel, the first step of the process.

2

Emotions Are Information

So, how *are* you feeling?

It's not a trick question. But it's more complicated than it sounds. We're always feeling something, usually more than one thing at a time. Our emotions are a continuous flow, not an occasional event. Inside each of us there's a river—placid and contained sometimes, but raging and overflowing its banks at others. There's a lot to navigate.

Picture yourself at the moment you awaken. Even then, as you slowly regain consciousness, you're feeling something. Perhaps you're desperate for another hour of rest. Or you feel supercharged and ready to vault out of bed. On a bad day, maybe it's dread at the thought of your commute or what you'll have to face at work in a few hours. It might be raining, which could dampen your mood even more. Or you could be feeling completely joyous and full of energy thanks to whatever it is you're going to do later. Maybe it's the great relief upon remembering that today is Saturday. Or the anticipation of a day that will be filled with creativity and excitement. Ten minutes from now, your emotional state might be completely different, depending on what you saw on the morning news, what your significant other told you about your plans for tonight, or what you just noticed about the shingles on the roof. Our emotional lives are a roller coaster, climbing high one moment and plunging the next.

Imagine how it must be for children. The same constant flow of feelings, running the gamut from crushingly negative to euphorically positive—from the moment they wake up in the morning, through the entire school day, to the moment they fall asleep. Except that children haven't learned yet how to manage their emotions—how to suppress and compartmentalize whatever's inconvenient at the moment, how to channel useful feelings for maximum benefit. They experience everything so intensely—boredom, frustration, anxiety, worry, excitement, elation. And they sit for hours in a classroom, expected to pay attention to every word spoken by a teacher who's probably under similar emotional pressures. Children's brains are less developed than ours, their defenses less robust, and yet the rivers of emotion that course through kids often are more powerful than the ones we experience. It's a wonder anybody learns anything.

So—a lot to contend with, second by second. We can't spend every minute focused on our emotions. We wouldn't have the time or attention to do much else. However, we can't go through life ignoring what we feel or minimizing its meaning. All emotions are an important source of information about what's going on inside us. Our multiple senses bring us news from our bodies, our minds, and the outside world, and then our brains process and analyze it and formulate our experience. We call that a *feeling*.

We humans have a long history of disregarding our feelings, however. It goes back millennia, even before the Stoic philosophers of ancient Greece argued that emotions were erratic, idiosyncratic sources of information. Reason and cognition were viewed as higher powers within us; once, the idea of "emotional intelligence" would have seemed inconceivable, a contradiction in terms. A great deal of Western literature, philosophy, and religion ever since has taught us that emotions are a kind of internal interference that gets in the way of sound judgment and rational thought. It's no coincidence that we still like to think of intelligence and emotion as coming from two completely separate parts of our bodies—one from the head, the other from the heart. Which of the two have we been taught to trust most?

Scientists didn't like emotions because, unlike intelligence, they can't be measured with standardized tests. IQ relies primarily on "cold" cognitive processes such as remembering a strand of digits or historical facts, while emotional intelligence relies on "hot" social-emotional-cognitive processes that are often highly charged, relationship driven, and focused on evaluating, predicting, and coping with feelings and behaviors—our own and other people's.

That's why the study of intelligence, formalized around 1900, continued the tradition of disregarding emotions. Throughout most of the twentieth century, psychologists and philosophers still debated whether emotions were associated in any way with logical thought and intelligent behavior. It's no wonder that the identification of an emotional intelligence occurred late compared with that of other kinds.

Then, in 1990, psychologists Peter Salovey and John Mayer introduced the first formal theory of emotional intelligence to the scientific literature. They defined it as "the ability to monitor one's own and others' feelings and emotions, to discriminate among them and to use this information to guide one's thinking and actions."

At Yale I interviewed Salovey, who said, "I started studying human emotions in a lab in college in the late 1970s. At that time, there wasn't much interest in emotions in psychology. The cognitive revolution was in full force and people viewed emotions as 'noise.' The idea was that we had emotions, but they didn't predict anything important. I just couldn't believe that was true, so I got very motivated to study emotions to show they mattered in a positive way. I wanted to show that we had an emotion system for a reason. We had an emotion system that helped us get through life."

Emotional intelligence was a synthesis of three burgeoning areas of scientific research, which demonstrated that emotions, when used widely, supported reasoning and complex problem solving.

First was the rediscovery of Charles Darwin's functional view of emotion. Back in the nineteenth century, he pioneered the idea that emotions signal valuable information and energize adaptive behavior central to survival. Fear finally got its due as being very useful indeed, especially in our species' early, threat-dense environments. Nothing like a good scare to get you up and fleeing a hungry saber-toothed cat.

Next came how emotions and moods play an essential role in thought processes, judgment, and behavior. Social scientists using clever experiments, and brain scientists who studied different brain regions, began to discover ways that emotions interact with cognition and behavior. Research showed that emotions give purpose, priority, and focus to our thinking. They tell us what to do with the knowledge that our senses deliver. They motivate us to act.

Psychologists proposed the idea of a "cognitive loop" that connects mood to judgment. For example, when a person is in a good mood, they're more likely to have positive thoughts and memories, which in turn keep the person thinking about positive things (the loop). In a classic study, psychologist Gordon Bower at Stanford University used hypnosis to make subjects feel happy or sad. Then they had to complete three tasks: recall lists of words, write entries in a diary, and remember experiences from childhood. Subjects who were made to feel sad recalled more negative memories and negative words and remembered more unpleasant events for their diaries. Likewise, the participants who were made to feel happy recalled happier memories and words and more positive events. Another study, by the late Alice Isen, a professor at Cornell University, and colleagues, showed some participants a comedy film and others no film at all and then tested them all for creative thinking. Results indicated a clear increase in creativity for those who saw the film—the ones in a "positive affect condition"—compared with the people in the other group. It's a natural bias—we all perceive and retrieve "mood-congruent" information most easily. It's just one of many ways that our emotions influence our thinking.

The third area of scientific inquiry was a search for "alternative" intelligences, to include a broad array of mental abilities rather than a single mental ability: IQ. There was increasing frustration among researchers with the inability of IQ tests to explain important life outcomes among individuals. Howard Gardner, a professor from Harvard University, proposed a theory of multiple intelligences that advised educators and scientists to place a greater emphasis on abilities beyond verbal and mathematical skills, such as intrapersonal (the awareness of one's own strengths and weaknesses) and interpersonal (the ability to communicate effectively and empathize with others) skills. Other researchers, including Robert Sternberg, a psychologist now at Cornell University, proposed a theory of "successful intelligence" and urged scientists and educators to consider creative and practical abilities. Nancy Cantor and John Kihlstrom, psychologists at Stanford University, built upon research in the 1920s by Edward Thorndike, pushing for a greater focus on "social intelligence"—the ability to accumulate knowledge about the social world, understand people, and act wisely in social relations.

By the late 1990s, emotional intelligence finally had achieved parity with the other forms of intelligence. Neuroscientists, psychologists, and intelligence researchers came to agree that emotion and cognition work hand in hand to perform sophisticated information processing. Research began to emerge that demonstrated there were individual differences in people's ability to reason with and about emotion. For example, research showed a wide range of skill in the abilities to perceive emotions accurately in facial expressions and regulate emotions.

Everything in this book is based on the past five decades of research into the roles—plural—that emotions play in our lives. At their highest level, from an evolutionary perspective, emotions have an extremely practical purpose: They ensure our survival. They make us smarter. If we didn't need them, they wouldn't exist.

I've championed five areas where our feelings matter most—the aspects of our everyday lives that are most influenced by our emotions. First, our emotional state determines where we direct our attention, what we remember, and what we learn. Second is decision making: when we're in the grip of any strong emotion—such as anger or sadness, but also elation or joy—we perceive the world differently, and the choices we make at that moment are influenced, for better or for worse. Third is our social relations. What we feel—and how we interpret other people's feelings—sends signals to approach or avoid, to affiliate with someone or distance ourselves, to reward or punish. Fourth is the influence of emotions on our health. Positive and negative emotions cause different physiological reactions within our bodies and brains, releasing powerful chemicals that, in turn, affect our physical and mental well-being. And the fifth has to do with creativity, effectiveness, and performance. In order to achieve big goals, get good grades, and thrive in our collaborations at work, we have to use our emotions as though they were tools. Which, of course, they are—or can be.

EMOTIONS AND ATTENTION, MEMORY, AND LEARNING

All learning has an emotional base.—PLATO

Let's start there, by examining how our emotions affect our attention and our memory, which together determine our ability to learn.

Think about it: emotions determine what you care about in the moment. If we're bored to tears or daydreaming about the coming weekend, we're not likely to absorb what we are reading on this page right now. If we're fearful, the source of that fear occupies all our thoughts.

If the house is on fire, we have but one goal: *Get me out of here!* If we're faced with sudden physical danger—whether we're out hiking and come face-to-face with a growling bear or we're strolling in the city at night and are stopped by an armed stranger—we've pretty much stopped thinking of anything else. Nature has wired our brains this way, and it's a good thing: any distraction in that moment could prove fatal.

Fear of intangible harm—of embarrassment, of shame, of looking foolish or inadequate in any way—works in a similar way. We may experience it as anxiety or worry instead of terror. The emotion may seem vain and irrational even to ourselves. Doesn't matter. As we've seen, feelings are highly impervious to cold logic. When we anticipate an unfavorable outcome under any circumstances, we're inhibited from thinking about much else. Perhaps our attention should be elsewhere, but we're helpless to redirect our minds at that moment.

Strong, negative emotions (fear, anger, anxiety, hopelessness) tend to narrow our minds—it's as though our peripheral vision has been cut off because we're so focused on the peril that's front and center. There's actually a physiological side to this phenomenon. When these negative feelings are present, our brains respond by secreting cortisol, the stress hormone. This inhibits the prefrontal cortex from effectively processing information, so even at a neurocognitive level our ability to focus and learn is impaired. To be sure, moderate levels of stress—feeling challenged—can enhance our focus. It's chronic stress that's toxic and makes it biologically challenging to learning. It's why I was a C student in middle school. I was too overwhelmed by family problems and bullying to be mentally present in class. When I was forty years old, I went to my hometown to visit the middle school I attended. Two unforgettable things happened. First, the moment I walked in I had a visceral reaction: I felt the fear and shame all over again. I immediately regressed to the fragile thirteen-year-old boy. Second, the only things I could remember were related to my bullying experiences. I couldn't remember most teachers' names or recall any subject matter I had learned.

It's not only negative feelings that can impair our mental capacity.

Let's say a high school student is in the grip of the typical hormonal hurricane that besets most teenagers. Romantic fantasies are fun to indulge, and world history can't be expected to compete. It's a wonder that adolescents manage to learn anything when you recall all the intoxicating daydreams that fill our heads at that age. Younger children are no less obsessed, but they're imagining the fun they'll have playing once the school day is through or going to Disney World for spring break. Joy and exuberance are as powerful as any other emotion when it comes to our ability to direct our thoughts where we want them to go. Instead of stimulating the production of cortisol, positive emotions are generally associated with the excretion of serotonin, dopamine, and other "feel-good" neurochemicals that exert their influence on thinking and behavior.

What research now shows is that different emotions serve different purposes for learning. If we need to engage our critical faculties—if, for instance, we have to edit a letter we've written and want to seek out flaws and correct any mistakes—a negative frame of mind might serve us better than its opposite. Pessimism can make it easier for us to anticipate things that could go wrong and then take the proper actions to prevent them. Guilt acts as a moral compass. Anxiety keeps us trying to improve things that a more generous mood might be willing to accept. Even anger is a great motivator—unlike resignation, it drives us to act and perhaps to fix what made us angry in the first place. If we're furious watching someone being mistreated, we're likely to step up and seek redress.

Imagine feeling smiley and bubbly, giddy with excitement, as you complete your final draft of a job application. It's possible, but it's a healthy fear, not joy, that can make us triple-check our punctuation and sentence structure. Negative emotions have a constructive function: they help narrow and focus our attention. It's sadness, not happiness, that can help us work through a difficult problem. It's excitement that stimulates lots of ideas. But too much enthusiasm won't bring needed consensus to a group—it will disperse the energy necessary for reasoning through the problem at hand, whether mathematical or interpersonal.

We're currently experiencing what seems like a crisis in education. Our students are tired, bored, and stressed. Their teachers are frustrated, pressured, and overwhelmed. Chronic disengagement and absenteeism are at record highs. How have we responded? By attempting to control student behavior even more than we already do. Or by introducing new math and literacy programs or instituting tougher learning standards. None of these solutions address the fact that how students feel is what gives meaning to what they are learning. The research is clear: emotions determine whether academic content will be processed deeply and remembered. Linking emotion to learning ensures that students find classroom instruction relevant. It's what supports students in discovering their purpose and passion, it's what drives their persistence.

Whenever we notice that we're suddenly having difficulty paying attention, or focusing, or remembering, we should ask ourselves: What emotion information is there, just beneath the surface of our thoughts? And what if anything can we do to regain a handle on our minds?

EMOTIONS AND DECISION MAKING

Affect is not just necessary for wisdom; it's also irrevocably woven into the fabric of every decision.
—ANTONIO DAMASIO, NEUROSCIENTIST,
UNIVERSITY OF SOUTHERN CALIFORNIA

Have you ever made a bad decision? You went with your gut, and when it turned out wrong you slapped your forehead and said, "Well, *that* was a dumb thing to do! What were you thinking?" It was a mental lapse or maybe just poor reasoning. In hindsight, it's plain to see what you failed to take into account. Let's just hope you learned a lesson.

A sensible thing to wish for—but what was the lesson?

We believe that our ability to reason and think rationally is our highest mental power, above our unruly emotional side. This is but a trick our brains play on us—in fact, our emotions exert a huge, though mostly unconscious, influence over how our minds function. This fact is especially evident when it comes to the decision-making process.

There are the obvious instances where emotion alone determines our actions. If we fear flying, we'll drive despite the increased danger. When we're overcome by passion, we might skip our usual measures to prevent unwanted pregnancy or sexually transmitted infections.

But emotion's influence extends far beyond that. Most decisions are attempts at predicting future outcomes: We ought to buy this house. I'm not going to take that job. Pasta is a great choice. In every case, we consider all the options and choose the one that seems most likely to result in a favorable outcome. In theory, at least.

In reality, our emotions largely determine our actions. If we're feeling something positive—confidence, optimism, contentment—we'll come to one conclusion about what we ought to do. If our emotions are negative—anxiety, anger, sadness—our decision may be quite different, even though we're working with the same set of facts.

The resulting patterns are fairly predictable. As discussed earlier in this chapter, anxiety narrows our attention and improves our focus on details. It makes us anticipate what could go wrong. That may not seem like a feeling we'd welcome, but it's a good frame of mind when we're performing tasks involving numbers, such as finances, for instance. If we're deciding whether to make an investment or a major purchase, a sunny mood might lead us to minimize the risks and do something we'll regret later. Negative emotions make us weigh facts carefully and err on the side of caution.

Positive emotions, on the other hand, fill us with the sense that life is going our way. If we're feeling strong, exuberant, energetic, we're more likely to base our decisions on heuristics—our gut instinct at that moment—than on careful reasoning. That's a useful outlook if we're planning a birthday party or when someone is in need of moral support, but maybe not so helpful when we're filing our tax return.

Emotion's true role in our decision making has been measured abundantly in experiments. Researchers will induce a mood in their subjects—by having them read or watch something happy or sad, for example—and then ask them to make decisions. In one study, subjects were seated in rooms that were either comfortable or uncomfortable and then asked about their satisfaction with their lives. The comfortable-room group reported being more satisfied. In a separate study, when subjects were made to feel sad, they perceived a mountain to be steeper than it actually was. And in a study on medical school admissions, it was found that applicants were more likely to be admitted on sunny days than when it rained (yes, admissions officers' decisions were biased by the weather!).

In an experiment we conducted at Yale, teachers were divided into two groups. One was told to remember and write about positive classroom experiences, and the other was assigned to recall a negative memory. Then all were asked to grade the same middle school essay. The positive-mood group marked the essay a full grade higher than the negative-mood group. When we asked the teachers if they believed their moods affected how they evaluated the papers, 87 percent said no. Judgments that entail a greater degree of subjectivity, such as grading a creative essay, are generally at a heightened risk of emotional bias compared with judgments that are more objective, such as grading a math test.

And our feelings can linger long past the moment that inspires them—influencing subsequent behavior without us knowing—it's known as "the incidental mood bias." So, for instance, if you argue with your kids over breakfast and are still angry while driving to work, you might drive more aggressively than usual and make risky decisions. When we recall happy moments from our past, we're likely to make decisions based in optimism and confidence. If we're remembering nega-tive things, we'll feel skeptical and pessimistic, and we'll decide things differently.

Anger's influence isn't what you might expect: researchers found that when people are angry, they tend to believe that individuals are at fault when things go wrong. When we're sad, we're more likely to blame external circumstances. Interestingly, anger makes people more optimistic than does sadness, possibly because angry people feel in greater control of their lives.

We make decisions continually, all day long, and most of them are small. We can't deliberate over each one, so we rely on our brains to make snap judgments. These issues come up all the time in con-temporary research into how our brains operate. There's the "thinking fast and thinking slow" concept, where our brains are believed to work on two separate but overlapping tracks, one that immediately responds without any or much deliberation and the other that takes its time and weighs the information first. When we use our brains for familiar or relatively simple functions, we come to quick responses, while novel situations or complex problems cause us to cogitate. These quick deci-sions are particularly susceptible to our moods and unconscious biases, especially when additional information is unavailable. We decide often with minimal conscious thinking.

None of this is to say that emotion inherently clouds our judgment. In fact, with greater emotional awareness, just the opposite may be true: our feelings can serve as another form of information, telling us important things about how we're responding to any given situation. When we are faced with a decision, anxiety may tell us one thing, en-thusiasm something completely different. Knowing this, we can take our emotional state into account before choosing a course of action. Is it our negative mood that's making us suspicious, or do we have a genu-ine reason to worry? Is our confidence a result of our exuberant mood, or is this truly the perfect decision?

EMOTION AND RELATIONSHIPS

No one cares how much you know, until
they know how much you care.
—THEODORE ROOSEVELT

Here's an experiment you can conduct using yourself as the guinea pig: Go through the list of everyone you encounter in the course of your daily life. Everybody—from your significant other and immediate family members to every co-worker, from the top to the bottom, every relative, friend, and acquaintance, the cashier at the supermarket, your doctor, your barber, the desk clerk at your gym, on and on. Just every human being whose path crosses yours, whether for hours on end or just five minutes.

Okay, now go through the list and ask yourself for your instant, top-of-the-head answer to this question: How do I feel when I encounter each and every one of them? How much do I look forward to my interactions with them all, individually? Do I smile at the thought of seeing this one or that? Does it leave me emotionally neutral? Or does something inside me tense up a little at the prospect? It doesn't have to be outright antipathy, just that little edge of anxiety knowing that this person and I will be face-to-face at some point.

What word would you use to describe the feeling you associate with each one? Is it anxiety? Joy? Confidence? Inadequacy? Boredom? Affection? Irritation? Those all make us more or less attractive to one another. Do you look forward to working alongside the colleague who's perpetually mad at the world?

Normally, this emotion isn't something we ever put into words or even think much about. It's like an instinctive reaction that comes from somewhere deeper than labels can easily express. Almost animalistic. When I see this person, something inside me leaps with joy. Or crashes in dejection. Or something in between.

Experiment over. Now perhaps you have a clearer notion of how

our strongest emotional reactions dictate the nature of all our relationships.

In seminars I conduct with teachers, I'll sometimes ask them to list
their students and consider the feeling that each name automatically
prompts. Is it love, dislike, trust, joy, fear, disgust? Next I'll say, Be
honest and think about how that emotion causes you to act toward
each of those children. I've had people break down crying during this
exercise. They instantly recognize how differently they treat each child
depending solely on their perception of how he or she makes them feel.
It has little to do with how the child performs in class, or the child's
needs, or anything they can name. It's just a strong, almost visceral reaction that usually has to do with something about the teacher, not the
student. These are mostly good teachers who do their best to treat each
student equally and want to establish a positive, nurturing relationship
with them all. But in the real world, despite all our best intentions, it
doesn't work that way. For some reason, teachers can barely make eye
contact with one child or give her or him focused attention, while they
eagerly look forward to interacting with other students and seek them
out during classroom activities.

Outside the classroom, we all operate in the same way. Human relations are infinitely complex because we ourselves are, but the basic dynamic is rather simple: approach or avoid. We tell people to come closer
or we tell them to back off. People communicate the same thing to us.
So much of what happens between human beings is a result of how we
communicate our emotions. And it all depends on something deep
inside us, perhaps hidden from our own view: our emotional state.

Relationships are the most important aspects of our lives. There's
plentiful scientific research showing the enormous influence they have
on our well-being—people with robust social networks enjoy better
mental and physical health and even live longer, while unfavorable outcomes are associated with a lack of connections to other people. The
purpose of relationships can be seen in all societies, even among animals: being surrounded by allies is a form of protection that can mean

the difference between life and death. Our need to attach ourselves to others isn't solely sentimental, even if it sometimes seems that way today.

Throughout this book, we will discuss all the ways we communicate our feelings about whomever we're dealing with at any given moment—the subtle, lightning-fast facial expressions, body language, vocal inflections, touch, and everything else in our arsenal of signals.

When we're expressing positive emotions authentically—contentment, compassion, joy—we do so in a way that draws in other people, whether it's your best friend or the supermarket cashier. They can read our signals clearly and may respond in kind, but that depends on *their* emotional state. People feeling emotions such as sorrow, shame, or anxiety often wish to discourage social interactions, and those signals are also being communicated. Those people might benefit most from engagement with others, but too often it's unlikely to happen. This is a particularly serious problem in our schools, which often reprimand children when they express a negative emotion rather than see it as a cry for help. These are the kids who are neglected, ignored, or suspended for misbehavior, when they should be given empathy, extra attention, and opportunities to build skills and meaningful relationships. Research shows that having just one caring adult can make the difference between whether a child will thrive or not.

We all have multitudes of relationships—with our children and parents and significant others, but also with the plumber, the driver in the next lane, our softball teammates, our boss or colleague, and the woman who holds the door open for us at the mall. And all these connections operate on the same basic principle: Our mood at any given moment is expressed in the signals we send out. If we're feeling joyful and open and expansive, it will make us confident and accepting of others. If we're feeling down on ourselves, it will color how we relate to other people—or if we connect at all. We tell people what we want from them by the messages we send, whether warm and hoping for a response in kind, or off-putting, when all we want is distance. This is the challenge for many people on the autism spectrum: they have difficulty reading the cues and coming up with a fitting response, and they have difficulty sending cues that other people understand. As a result, they struggle building and maintaining relationships.

We also express emotions in order to get what we want from the people in our lives. If we make a show of anger, we may not earn much empathy, but we instill fear in others and maybe remove any obstacles that were in our way. If, on the other hand, we need cooperation and understanding, we know what emotion message to send that will get the response we desire.

People feeling compassion see greater common humanity with strangers. They punish others less, are more generous and cooperative, and are willing to sacrifice for others. Research shows that high-powered individuals tend to be less responsive to the emotions of people around them. In one study, these individuals responded with less compassion than people with less power when listening to someone describe suffering. Does this phenomenon explain anything about our political and business leaders?

Sometimes the emotions we feel send signals that elicit the opposite of the response we want and need. Picture a typical child: if he's troubled or anxious, he may wish that his parent or teacher would reach out and offer comfort. But when those adults sense that child's emotional state, especially when he's "acting out," they may respond in just the opposite way, because of their own emotional response to the signals of a negative mood. This dynamic rules much of human interaction—when we need emotional support most is when we're least likely to receive it.

I remember being in seventh-grade math class, where two students would regularly write all over a jacket I wore each day. I'm certain I wore that jacket as a form of protection. My fear and despair had to show in my face, body, and chronic disengagement. But the teacher didn't intervene. What was his mindset? Stay away—this kid's a wimp who needs to toughen up? Was he too preoccupied with his own issues to pay attention to mine? Perhaps he was just at a loss about what to do. Either way, I suffered socially, emotionally, and academically.

There was a great moment in the film *Broadcast News* where a character asks, "Wouldn't this be a great world if insecurity and desperation made us more attractive? If 'needy' was a turn-on?" Unfortunately, we humans don't work that way (yet).

EMOTIONS AND HEALTH

Emotional sickness is avoiding reality at any cost.
Emotional health is facing reality at any cost.
—M. SCOTT PECK

You lie awake at three A.M., staring at the ceiling, anxious about some serious problem. Impossible to sleep. We've all been there. You're too pressured and distracted to even think about working out, and besides, you have too much else on your plate, so you skip the gym, even though you know it makes you feel good to go. Can't be helped. Meals are erratic. Instead of thinking about dinner and planning to shop and cook, you grab a pizza on the way home from work. It's been happening a lot lately. And after that's done, you need to decompress, so it's a pint of ice cream in front of the TV for an hour. Until it's finally time for bed and another three A.M. staring at the ceiling. . . .

For a moment, forget about your emotional health—imagine what you're doing to your physical health.

When considering the influence of emotion on our well-being, we must first remember that our brains—where most of our feelings originate—are as much a part of our bodies as any other organ, fed by the same flow of blood, oxygen, and nutrients. Our emotions are linked to physiological reactions in our brains, releasing hormones and other powerful chemicals that, in turn, affect our physical health, which has an impact on our emotional state. It's all connected.

That's why physical sickness can be caused by a mind under emotional stress. But there's also the opposite phenomenon: physical wellness that's fostered by positive feelings. Both kinds underscore the importance of managing our emotional lives.

Even our *mindset* about stress can influence health outcomes, from weight loss to insomnia. In one study, Alia Crum, an assistant professor at Stanford University, randomly assigned three hundred employees at a finance company to watch two different three-minute videos about stress. Half of the participants watched a video that reinforced the negative aspects of stress; the others watched a similar video, but the messaging reinforced the positive side. After four weeks, the employees were surveyed: the "stress is bad" group experienced more negative health symptoms than those in the "stress is good" group.

Inside our brains, hormones and other neurochemicals are being turned on and off depending on what we're feeling at any given moment. The hypothalamic-pituitary-adrenal (HPA) axis, located in the midbrain, is one of the major neuroendocrine systems that controls how we respond to stress and also regulates emotions and moods. The HPA axis is where certain hormones, such as adrenaline and cortisol, originate. Researchers studying this region of the brain have found that early-life exposure to mild, everyday stressors enhances our future ability to regulate emotions and confers lifelong resilience. But exposure to extreme or prolonged stress does just the opposite—it induces hyperactivity in the HPA axis and lifelong susceptibility to stress.

The difference between good stress and bad stress mainly has to do with duration and intensity. For instance, having to prepare a compelling presentation for a client is a form of stress, but the good kind. It's caused by the challenge of achieving a desired goal and lasts only a short time. The ending of a game, or a major event such as a wedding day, affects us similarly. Stress inducing but happy. These events prompt the momentary release of stress hormones, but then it ends. Research at the Stanford University School of Medicine found that short bouts of stress can boost immunity and raise levels of cancer-fighting molecules—and the effect lasts for weeks after the stressful situation ends.

We have evolved to handle short-term stress—hormones are released, allowing us to respond successfully to the crisis, and then turn off at the tap. That's not what happens at some workplaces, where we may be forced to endure eight hours daily with a boss who makes life a living hell, or at schools where students may dread the bullies on the bus ride home. Many of us spend hours and entire days under emotional duress, until it becomes a chronic condition. Our brains are bathed in a constant flow of stress hormones, for which evolution has definitely not prepared us. We don't suffer only emotionally in those instances—our physical health is affected too.

"Stress leaves you in a fight-or-flight state in which your body turns off long-term building and repair projects," said Robert Sapolsky, a professor at Stanford University, in his book *Behave*. "Memory and accuracy are impaired. You tire more easily, you can become depressed and reproduction gets downgraded."

There's ample scientific evidence of the long-term harm caused by childhood emotional trauma, such as bullying. Children may experience compromised immunity to disease, digestive tract pain and upset, headaches, poor sleep, inability to concentrate, and depression. These effects can persist into adulthood, creating physical and mental health problems long after the bullying is in the past.

Feeling "down"—pessimism, apathy, depression—is linked to low levels of serotonin and dopamine, the so-called feel-good neurotransmitters. Serotonin plays a role in pain perception, which may be why people experiencing negative emotions report more severe symptoms of illness, and nearly half of patients with depression also suffer aches and pains.

Negative emotional states—anxiety, anger, sadness, stress—are closely associated with unhealthy behaviors, such as poor diet, smoking, excessive drinking, physical inactivity, and social isolation, many of which we found in a recent study with more than five thousand teachers from across the United States. Those are the same lifestyle factors that contribute to our most feared and widespread illnesses: heart disease, cancer, type 2 diabetes, addiction, dementia. These conditions in turn have a devastating impact on our emotional lives, and the feedback loop turns into a downward spiral for our health, mental and physical. Ultimately, they deepen our feelings of hopelessness and despair that we will ever manage to improve our moods or our health. Interestingly, we found that a positive workplace climate acted as a buffer for the deleterious effects of negative emotions on health outcomes for teachers.

There's a great deal of medical research linking hostility and anger to heart disease. Men reporting the highest levels of anger were over two and a half times more likely to suffer cardiac events such as heart attack than other men. Negative emotions have been associated with hypertension, increased heart rate, constriction of peripheral blood vessels, unhealthy blood lipids, and decreased immune system function.

Not only does an angry outburst cause a spike in blood pressure, but every time we recall what made us so mad, our blood pressure rises again. According to one study, a thirty-minute argument with your significant other can slow your body's ability to heal by at least a day. And if you argue regularly, that delay is doubled. Even subtle forms of anger, such as impatience, irritability, and grouchiness, may damage health.

We can see the influence of our emotions on our physical health in less dire ways too. The stress associated with knowing you have to deliver a speech can double the severity of allergy symptoms for two days. Feeling sad makes symptoms of illness seem more severe and cause greater discomfort. In one study, people who scored low on positive emotions were three times as likely to become sick after exposure to a virus than those who scored higher. When the latter group did get sick, their symptoms were less severe.

But our emotions can also prompt the release of beneficial neuro-chemicals and hormones. Crying is soothing because it carries stress hormones out of our bodies. Feelings of gratitude increase oxygen levels in our tissues, speed healing, and boost our immune system. Being in love was found to raise the level of nerve growth factor, a hormone-like substance that restores the nervous system and improves memory. The effect lasts for about a year, according to researchers. In one study, laughter caused by watching a comedy film increased the flow of beta-endorphins, which enhance our mood, and stimulated growth hormones, which repair our cells. Even the anticipation of laughter was found to lower the levels of cortisol and adrenaline. Laughter may also reduce the risk of heart attack. Feeling good, therefore, may encourage healthy behaviors, which in turn can promote greater emotional well-being and physical health.

In the wake of the September 11, 2001, attacks, U.S. college students were tested, and those who experienced the most positive emotions—gratitude, love, and so forth—were less likely to develop depressive symptoms later on. This suggests that after a crisis, people who have more positive feelings may be more resilient than those who experience fewer positive emotions.

We'll never eradicate negative emotions from our lives or those of our kids. Nor should we. But we need to attend to the play of positive and negative emotions, which is out of balance for too many of us. As we reported earlier, our research at Yale revealed that high school students, teachers, and business professionals experience negative emotions up to 70 percent of the time they are in school or at work. Their feelings aren't the only thing at stake—so is their health. What will it take to switch the ratio of negative-to-positive emotions? What's your ratio?

EMOTIONS AND CREATIVITY

Rational thoughts never drive people's
creativity the way emotions do.
—NEIL DEGRASSE TYSON

Many of us need to feel creative in order to feel alive, engaged, and fully involved in life and whatever it throws at us. Otherwise we're just treading water. But what do we mean by creativity?

There's the obvious answer—artistic work such as painting, music, literature, and the professions that demand (and reward) creativity, such as architecture, science, design, and engineering, among others.

But creativity is much more universal than that. It's an important element of every human life. Whenever we make a decision or face a challenge, we have an opportunity to be creative—to respond to the moment in a way that doesn't just repeat what's always been done before (and perhaps always failed before too). Daily, each of us has many chances to be creative, to act in new and thoughtful ways. It's what makes life an adventure.

But there can be something scary about creativity too. It represents a break with the status quo and a step into the unknown. Creative decisions, even in the smallest matters, are a way of saying we think we have a better idea. And then comes the feedback—from others, but even from ourselves: What if your new way doesn't work out so well? What if you've made things worse (at least in somebody's eyes, though maybe not yours)? What makes you think you're so creative anyway? You can see that our creative impulses and our emotions are closely intertwined.

Many of us believe that personality and intelligence alone drive our ability to be creative. Or that creativity is an all-or-nothing gift, rather than a set of skills that can be improved with practice. True, some personality traits such as "openness to experience" are reliably related to it, but traits alone don't account for everything. And research confirms that creativity is only modestly associated with IQ (meaning you don't have to be a genius to be creative!).

This is where our emotional lives extend even beyond the personal. Creativity is the lifeblood of our culture and our economy. In a poll, fifteen hundred corporate CEOs said that an employee's creativity was the single best indicator of future success. Without innovation, societies stagnate and die.

Creativity also includes two other factors: performance and effectiveness. Creativity can't exist only in the abstract, in our minds and nowhere else. That's just having a rich imagination! The creative process needs to be followed by concrete action. Once we devise new strategies, we must have the confidence to put them to use. Effective performance is as much a part of creativity as the initial, animating idea.

But whether we take advantage of all the possibilities every time is a different matter. Safe to say, at times we all *feel* less creative than we'd like to be. That's because our creativity is so closely tied to our emotional state—even though the connection may not be so obvious.

Again and again, in working with educators, families, and children, we wind up discussing the ubiquitous problems of stress and frustration—the despair of feeling as though we lack the power to make meaningful changes for the better. It's hard to imagine a worse feeling. For a child, it can be devastating—children have little control over their lives under the best of conditions. We all go through tough times, but most of us believe that if we persevere, we can find solutions. That's another form of creativity: everyday creativity, the ability to keep discovering new answers when the old ones no longer work. What must life be like for the children and adults who can't hope even for that?

We can see how it plays out in schools. Kyung Hee Kim, a professor at the School of Education at the College of William & Mary, made extensive studies of creativity among schoolchildren and found that it has been in decline for the past two decades. Her conclusions are based on results from the Torrance Tests of Creative Thinking (TTCT), which measure creativity, defined as the ability to respond to situations in ways that are novel and original. For example, people could be asked for all the possible uses for a paper clip or the consequences of people becoming invisible at will. She examined normative data for the TTCT through time, from kindergarten to senior year of high school, and writes, "Children have become less emotionally expressive, less energetic, less talkative and verbally expressive, less humorous, less imaginative, less unconventional, less lively and passionate, less perceptive, less apt to connect seemingly irrelevant things, less synthesizing, and less likely to see things from a different angle." Who or what could we blame except parents and an educational system that often squash original thinking and penalize students for using their imagination? Our students get the message rather quickly from our obsession with kindergarten "readiness," to society's detriment. Interestingly, when the developer of the creativity test, Dr. E. Paul Torrance, administered it to students and then tracked them years into the future, he found that scores on his famous creativity tests were a better predictor of adult creative achievements than IQ.

When discussing creative thinking, psychologists often use the terms *convergent* and *divergent* thinking. The former operates when searching for only one correct solution to a problem or only one proper answer to a question and tries to arrive at it by mostly straight-ahead, linear thinking. The divergent approach moves in all directions—it assumes there are many possible solutions and tries to consider each, especially the most creative, unusual ones.

The impulse to create seems to come naturally to the human brain. However, we must be encouraged to express it. In schools, it's hard to be creative when convergent thinking—the ability to remember facts and perform well on standardized tests—is most highly rewarded. To engage children and prepare them for the workforce, they must be given more opportunities and encouragement to be creative. For that to happen, schools need to restructure learning so that it promotes unconventional thinking and fresh approaches to problem solving across content areas, not just in the arts. For example, more and more schools are incorporating project-based learning and design thinking—a five-stage process for solving complex problems that includes (1) defining a problem; (2) understanding the human needs involved; (3) reframing the problem in human-centric ways; (4) generating a multitude of ideas; and (5) a hands-on approach in prototyping and testing.

Research shows that divergent thinking results in feelings of joy, pride, and satisfaction. A study across five countries with four different languages found that working on creative tasks leads to an increase in positive emotions and autonomy. Another study showed that creative behavior on a given day leads to more positive emotions and a sense of flourishing the next day. As with so much about our emotional lives, there's a feedback loop at work: feeling good encourages us to act creatively, which makes us feel even better.

But happiness is not the single key to creativity. In fact, modest levels of stress have been found in some cases to significantly improve creative performance compared with no stress at all. Even emotions such as anger and distress can serve as motivation for creative thinking and enhance creativity. Take the high school students in Parkland, Florida. They have channeled their anger about the horrific school shooting to build a persuasive campaign around gun reform. The role of sympathy in creative thinking has also been explored. College students were induced to feel sympathy through a slide show of distressed elderly adults, then asked to generate ideas and design a floor plan for an office reception area to make it more welcoming to the elderly. Compared with the control group, the "sympathy" participants showed greater originality in thinking. One explanation is that sympathy is a reaction to other people's suffering and therefore produces intrinsic motivation to generate solutions that reduce their distress.

Creativity is especially important in the face of adversity—when we're disappointed because plan A didn't work out; when we tried hard and still received negative feedback; when someone stands in the way of our progress or even tries to prevent it. We first have to manage our hurt or anger—not deny it but accept it and then put it to good use, as a motivational force. That's where our creativity can come to our rescue and allow us to achieve our goal despite obstacles.

According to my colleague at Yale, Zorana Ivcevic Pringle, a creativity researcher, "Emotions are both the spark that fires the engine of creativity and the fuel that keeps the firing burning when other people try to douse it, or the kindling runs low." Emotions rule the whole creative process, from motivating creative work to idea generation to persisting toward the actualization of our own ideas. It's the challenge that keeps us striving.

Now do you see how complex that simple question "How do you feel?" really can be? That emotional roller coaster is no small matter—it has an enormous influence over the most important areas of our lives. Religious leaders, poets, and playwrights have known this for centuries; over the past few decades, the scientists have begun to catch up. Now we know better than the ancients (and not so ancients) the degree to which emotions guide everything else. That's the first step toward accepting who we truly are. What, then, is the next step?

3

How to Become an Emotion Scientist

HOW ARE YOU FEELING right now? Can you be sure?

That may seem like a ridiculous question—of course we all know exactly what we're feeling. It may be the only thing about which we can be certain.

So if it's all so completely, effortlessly self-evident, why would we need a science of emotion and emotional intelligence? We speak of emotion skills, but doesn't that mean there is something to be learned—or not? Indeed it does: it's a safe bet that no one in the history of the human race has ever known precisely what she or he is feeling, in all its complexity and contradiction and chaos, at all times. Our neurons are firing hundreds of times a second, and lots of what goes on up there is pure, roiling emotion.

Scientists refer to intelligences as hot or cold, hot being the emotional one and cold, of course, the rational one.

But they don't take turns operating. If I'm computing what I owe in taxes, I'm using cold intelligence, though my reasoning powers will absolutely be affected if five minutes ago I noticed a weird lump on my dog's neck or I had an argument with my next-door neighbor. We have one brain made up of several regions, each with its own functions, and sometimes they pull us in different directions.

Given all that, how could anyone *but* a scientist make sense of it? That's why we all must strive to become emotion scientists.

You could be brilliant, with an IQ that Einstein would envy, but if you're unable to recognize your emotions and see how they're affecting your behavior, all that cognitive firepower won't do you as much good as you might imagine. A gifted child who doesn't have the permission to feel, along with the vocabulary to express those feelings and the ability to understand them, won't be able to manage complicated emotions around friendships and academics, limiting his or her potential.

As we saw in the previous chapter, our most important mental functions have an emotional aspect, even if they seem to be purely in the realm of "cognition." And those factors determine significant real-life outcomes—our relationships, our performance, our decision making, even our physical health. Our feelings encourage us to treat the people we care about with love and respect or disregard their needs and wishes; help us focus our thinking or distract us; fill us with enthusiasm and energy or deplete our will; open us up to the outside world or wall us off from it. Feelings motivate us to do things that improve our lives and those of the people around us, but they can also adversely influence our actions—without us even realizing it. In fact, that's when we're most vulnerable to emotion's impact: when we fail to detect it.

When we are making a decision, there are two kinds of emotions: *integral* and *incidental*. Integral emotions are directly caused by the action at hand—we're fearful while climbing a tricky mountain path; we're joyful as we're falling in love. All completely understandable and connected to the moment. Incidental emotions have nothing to do with what's going on—as we described earlier, we had an argument with our kids, and our lingering feelings of frustration and anger influence how we drive to work or interact with colleagues at the office. These are the emotions that infiltrate our thinking without us being aware.

Only by becoming emotion scientists will we learn the skills to use our emotions wisely. Not suppress them or ignore them—in fact, just the opposite. We'll no longer be controlled by feelings we may not even perceive. We'll also be able to help the people we interact with—loved ones, colleagues—manage theirs.

Knowing what emotions tell us is the first, necessary part of the process. For example, anxiety is a signal that we feel something important is beyond our control. Fear or uneasiness can make us risk-averse. That can be a positive thing—it may steer us away from taking foolish chances. But if we're too risk-averse, or give up in the face of obstacles too easily, we'll never try anything, thereby guaranteeing failure. That's why we need to understand our emotions, be aware of how they influence our actions, and have strategies to regulate them.

Becoming an emotion scientist will help us to recognize the physical symptoms that sometimes accompany strong feelings. Suddenly I'm feverish and my heart is racing; or I'm feeling a queasy ache in my stomach. All real sensations, sometimes emotional rather than physiological, sometimes not. Lisa Feldman Barrett, a professor at Northeastern University, recently shared with me that when our "body budget" is running low and we feel distressed, our brains search around for things that might be wrong in our lives to make sense of the distress. When these symptoms present themselves, we don't always pause to ask: Is there an emotion behind this, and what can I do about it? Or am I just dehydrated or hungry or tired and need to drink or eat something or just go to bed?

An emotion scientist has the ability to pause even at the most stressful moments and ask: What am I reacting to? We can learn to identify and understand all our feelings, integral and incidental, and then respond in helpful, proportionate ways—once we acquire emotion skills. But what exactly are they?

In 1990, Peter Salovey and John Mayer published a landmark paper, "Emotional Intelligence," in a little-known journal (after it was rejected by multiple top-tier publications). That article has since served as the academic foundation for most research into emotional intelligence. In it, they asserted that the majority of life tasks are influenced by emotion. We all have emotion skills, the authors wrote, but to varying degrees. And we can all increase our emotional intelligence, which Salovey and Mayer defined as

> the ability to perceive accurately, appraise, and express emotion; the ability to access and/or generate feelings when they facilitate thought; the ability to understand emotion and emotional knowledge; and the ability to regulate emotions to promote emotional and intellectual growth.

That's a fine textbook definition. We should all possess those skills. But it's hard to infer what emotional intelligence looks like in practice from that definition alone. There are individual differences in how we process information of every type. Some of us are naturally better at math than others, while some of us excel at language-based tasks. But we all learn and improve in those areas. Similarly, some of us are more fluent and intuitive than others when it comes to emotional matters. But we can all learn and improve here too.

In my seminars, I often ask people to describe an emotionally intelligent person. Try it yourself now: What are the skills?

Some people say *empathy*, which allows us to relate to what others are feeling. Empathy is about having a shared emotional experience. If you feel shame from childhood experiences, and I've also experienced shame, then we can feel empathy for each other. Empathy often is enriched with emotion skills. Empathy can help you connect with someone, but it won't necessarily help you to support a person in managing his or her difficult emotion or stop you from getting lost in someone else's shoes. That's where emotion skills come into play.

Neither is what we commonly think of as *emotional stability*. We tend to view a calm, poised demeanor as a sign of superior emotional wisdom. It denotes inner peace and harmony. People who are serene and "together" may possess great emotion skills, but the same may be true of those who are conspicuously neurotic. In fact, sometimes—out of pure necessity—people who are high in neuroticism also demonstrate great emotion skills. They need them in order to regulate their own tumultuous inner lives. But neither stability nor neuroticism equals emotional intelligence.

Grit, which Angela Duckworth, a professor at the University of Pennsylvania, defines as "perseverance and passion for long-term goals," has become a popular psychological construct in recent years. Research shows that grit is associated with many important outcomes from academic achievement to income. But grit isn't an emotion skill. There are plenty of gritty people who struggle with regulating their emotions. Grit and emotional intelligence are not in competition with each other but rather work hand in hand to support people in achieving their goals. Here's how: On the path to success, gritty people (like myself) often fail to achieve certain goals; we get frustrated, disappointed, or overwhelmed and receive negative feedback. Therefore, having a repertoire of emotion-regulation strategies can help gritty people to overcome difficult emotions and obstacles that arise on the journey toward achieving long-term goals. And as we know, the right amount of persistence may lead to success, but too much can be counterproductive. I've had my share of students who, emboldened by the belief in the power of grit, go so far overboard that they undermine their own best efforts owing to their lack of social awareness.

Resilience also is mentioned as an emotion skill. According to the American Psychological Association, it is "the process of adapting well in the face of adversity, trauma, tragedy, threats or significant sources of stress—such as family and relationship problems, serious health problems or workplace and financial stressors." Research by Tom Boyce from the University of California–San Francisco and colleagues has revealed biological markers that differentiate how "sensitive" children (referred to as "orchids") respond to environmental changes compared with how "resilient" children (who they call "dandelions") react. Dandelion children may thrive in most any condition, whereas orchid children tend to be more fearful and overwhelmed in uncertain social situations. Whether an orchid or a dandelion child does better or worse likely has to do with how families, teachers, and peers support their emotional development. If neglected, orchid children promptly wither—but if they are raised in supportive conditions, they not only survive but flourish compared with dandelion children. Emotion skills are likely the antecedent to building resilience.

Finally, emotion skills are not a constellation of traits, such as confidence or charisma or popularity. It doesn't mean having a "good" personality, whatever that is. It isn't kindness or warmth or high self-esteem. It isn't optimism. Those may all be desirable qualities that make us appealing to the rest of the world. We may aspire to any or all of the above. But they're not emotion skills.

So, what are they? First, emotion skills must be acquired. Nobody is born with them all in place and ready to work. Emotion skills amplify our strengths and help us through challenges. If I'm an extrovert and need to shine, then I must learn to read my environment, so I can see when I overwhelm others and tone myself down. If I'm an introvert, my tendency to be quiet and subdued might underwhelm people at home, school, or the workplace, so I will need to amp myself up at times, so the world can see my enthusiasm.

Over the years, I've run into some strange ideas about emotional intelligence and its purposes. Once, during a seminar I led at a major tech company, a top executive took issue with the idea that he had anything to learn. "I want you to teach the people who work for me to learn how to deal with *my* emotions," he said.

At a conference for intellectually gifted individuals, where I was a presenter, people were wearing name tags with colored dots. When I asked my host what the colors meant, she said that green indicated "I'm comfortable with receiving a hug," yellow meant "Ask before hugging," and red proclaimed "Stay away!" That was the first (and only) conference I've attended where people publicly announced their comfort levels around emotion and physical contact. It also was my first "on-the-scene learning" experience that supported the empirical research I had done, which demonstrated the small correlation between emotional intelligence and IQ.

Another time, at a demanding medical school, a senior professor made little effort to hide his skepticism. When I asked if there were any questions, he stood up and said, "What happened to academia? We are training future Nobel laureates here, not nice people." As if the two qualities couldn't coexist within one person. There were so many prejudices, weaknesses, and contradictions encoded into that statement, it would have taken many hours of discussion (and probably a lot of therapy) to untangle it all. The plainest, shortest response I had was, "Well, you *could* be training a lot *more* Nobel laureates if . . ." (I later asked the chair of the department, "Is this really happening?" He whispered, "Why do you think I brought you in?")

To some observers, emotional intelligence or emotion skills signify something fuzzy and touchy-feely, like a retreat from reality. This is especially so in the business world. In fact, just the opposite is true. These are mental skills like any others—they enable us to think smarter, more creatively, and to get better results from ourselves and the people around us. There's nothing squishy about that. Emotional intelligence doesn't allow feelings to get in the way—it does just the opposite. It restores balance to our thought processes; it prevents emotions from having undue influence over our actions; and it helps us to realize that we might be feeling a certain way for a reason.

For more than twenty years, our team has synthesized research in psychology, education, and neuroscience in order to teach the emotion skills necessary for children and adults to thrive. These abilities represent the principal aspects of emotion knowledge, competencies, and processes found in the psychological literature on emotional development and intelligence. Based on that, we've developed an approach for making emotion skills an integral part of education for leaders, managers, teachers, students, and families. It's being used all over the world, in school systems, in corporations, and in other institutions.

Throughout the rest of this book, we'll explore those skills in detail. Here, I'll provide a brief introduction. They're known by an acronym—RULER.

The first skill: Recognizing the occurrence of an emotion—by noticing a change in one's own thoughts, energy, or body or in someone else's facial expression, body language, or voice. That's the first clue that something important is happening.

The second skill: Understanding, which means that we know the cause of emotions and see how they influence our thoughts and decisions. This helps us make better predictions about our own and others' behavior.

The third skill: Labeling, which refers to making connections between an emotional experience and the precise terms to describe it. People with a more mature "feelings vocabulary" can differentiate among related emotions such as pleased, happy, elated, and ecstatic. Labeling emotions accurately increases self-awareness and helps us to communicate emotions effectively, reducing misunderstanding in social interactions.

The fourth skill: Expressing, which means knowing how and when to display our emotions, depending on the setting, the people we're with, and the larger context. People who are skilled in this area understand that unspoken rules for emotional expression, also called "display rules," often direct the best way to express what they feel and modify their behaviors accordingly.

The fifth skill: Regulating, which involves monitoring, tempering, and modifying emotional reactions in helpful ways, in order to reach personal and professional goals. This doesn't mean ignoring inconvenient emotions—rather, it's learning to accept and deal with them. People with this skill employ strategies to manage their own emotions and help others with theirs.

In the RULER framework, the first three skills—Recognizing, Understanding, and Labeling—help us to accurately identify and decode what we and others are feeling. Then, the two remaining skills—

Expressing and Regulating—tell us how we can manage those emotions to achieve desired outcomes—our ultimate goal.

Research on general intelligence, or IQ, dates back to the early 1900s. Part of the reason the concept of emotional intelligence lags behind that of IQ is that there are reliable, scientifically proven tests to measure the latter. A licensed psychologist will charge a couple thousand dollars to administer a standardized three-hour examination that produces a defining number: your intelligence quotient. IQ has been with us for more than a century. No such comprehensive evaluation exists—yet—for emotional intelligence. Without a precise measure, we find it easy to dismiss it as a subjective, imprecise notion.

Daily life requires emotion skills at every turn yet provides little reliable feedback on how well we're doing or if we're improving. Few institutions of learning devote any time to teaching or assessing emotion skills. We're still in the beginning stages of unpacking emotion science, including how best to measure and teach the skills. Think about it: How much formal instruction, at home or at school, did you receive in the five key emotion areas described above? If you're like most of us, not much.

Yet I am comfortable making the case that emotional intelligence is as important as IQ. We know for a fact that no matter how smart you are, your emotions will have an influence—positive or negative—on your rational thought processes. That's important.

We've already explained the five key emotion skills, so let's try an experiment: a simple self-test you can take to measure your own. You'll have to score yourself from 1 (very unskilled) to 5 (very skilled) on five statements that neatly sum up what it takes to be an emotion scientist:

- I am able to accurately recognize my own and others' emotions.
- I am aware of the causes and consequences of my own and others' feelings.

- I have a refined emotion vocabulary.
- I am skilled at expressing the full range of emotions.
- I am skilled at managing my own emotions and at helping others manage theirs.

Okay, what was your score? A 25 is perfect and a 5 is the worst you can do.

How confident are you in the significance of your score? Let's admit the fatal flaw in this test: none of us is completely unbiased when it comes to estimating our own mental skills, emotional or otherwise. In a study we conducted of college students, we asked how they thought they would perform on the standardized emotional intelligence assessment compared with their roommates and all other undergraduates at the university. Nearly 80 percent of the students believed they would perform above the fiftieth percentile. So clearly we're inclined to overstate our emotion skills. Perhaps unsurprising, male students' estimates of their scores were significantly higher than those of the women, despite the fact that the men did worse than the women when they took a performance-based test.

It's possible to go online and find many similar self-tests that purport to quickly and accurately measure emotional intelligence. Like the one we just took, these are mostly superficial and misleading, often measuring personality traits rather than emotion skills and reflecting the universal desire to feel superior to our fellow human beings when it comes to the wisdom of the heart.

In the corporate world, emotional intelligence is regularly assessed using a "360-degree" format for the purposes of promotion or executive coaching. In this case, a person's score is based on his or her own self-report *in addition* to evaluations provided by peers, subordinates, and supervisors. These assessments are mostly concerned with self-control, trustworthiness, conscientiousness, adaptability, teamwork ability, the ability to influence others, and inspirational leadership—all potentially important aspects of being a good leader and manager. The general consensus among researchers is that these tools measure perceived traits, competencies, and aspects of one's reputation, but not emotion skills.

For the reasons stated above, there is a general agreement in psychology that performance tests (as opposed to self-report scales) are the gold standard, because they measure actual capacity for mental tasks. In regard to emotional intelligence, Salovey and Mayer, along with David Caruso, cofounder of Emotional Intelligence Skills Group, developed a performance test. It endeavors to measure how well people perform tasks and solve emotion-laden problems. The test has been an important tool for research purposes, but even the most sophisticated test can't predict how someone would respond in real-life situations where emotion skills are required. The real test of emotion skills isn't while reading on the beach; it's when someone kicks sand in your face! Currently, our team is working with Professor Sigal Barsade at the Wharton School, University of Pennsylvania, to build a suite of dynamic performance tests of emotional intelligence to capture emotion skills in real time.

There's another reason why defining emotional intelligence is so elusive: the lack of clear terminology. Most of us use words such as "emotion" and "feeling" more or less interchangeably, with a general understanding of what they mean. But there are some subtle and important distinctions too. Let's go through the glossary.

An *emotion*—happy, sad, angry—arises from an appraisal of an internal or external stimulus. By appraisal I mean an interpretation of what is happening in the world or my mind through the lens of my present goals or concerns. We hear, see, feel (through touch), taste, or smell something that alerts us to a shift in the environment. We are provoked by a memory or sensation, or an event, something someone says or does, or something we witness or experience. I think about someone who treated me unfairly or someone actually treats me unfairly, and I feel angry.

Emotions are mostly short-lived (have you ever felt surprised for an hour?). They usually include a physiological reaction, such as a blush, chills, or an increased heart rate, and a release of neurochemicals to prepare you for action. They are often expressed automatically in our facial expressions, body language, and other nonverbal cues. Emotions also are accompanied by a subjective experience in our conscious minds. When we feel happy we have positive thoughts. Being upset turns us into pessimists. Finally, emotions mobilize us into action—to approach or avoid, fight or flee.

The classical view of emotions was that they were evolutionary adaptations and that people across all cultures experienced and displayed the same basic emotions in the same ways. For example: We developed the feeling of fear because it was advantageous to our survival, and we all express it in the same way because it is part of our biological nature.

Today, our understanding has become more nuanced. Recent research emphasizes that emotions are fully intertwined not only with our biology but also with our individual life experiences and culture. We don't all fear the same things, and we don't all express joy in the same ways. When schoolchildren in the United States are asked to draw a happy face, it sports a huge smile. When Asian children are given the same task, the smiles are smaller. This doesn't mean they are less happy than their American counterparts, only that perhaps they experience and express their happiness differently. As we mature, our emotional repertoire becomes more precise (one hopes). Preschoolers have one word for angry: mad. Older children in schools where we work learn to make fine distinctions, using concepts such as annoyed, aggravated, irritated, livid, and enraged.

A *feeling* is our internal response to an emotion. I'm angry about something that's happening between us, it's caused me to give up hope, and I can't keep going this way. That's a feeling. It's nuanced, subtle, multidimensional. When you ask someone how they're feeling, the answer is sometimes an emotion, such as happy, sad, afraid, angry. But they may also say they're feeling supported, connected, valued, respected, and appreciated. These words do not refer to emotions per se but are motivational and relationship states that are steeped in emotion. Technically, an athlete doesn't *feel* motivated to run a marathon; it's the athlete's current and anticipated feelings of joy and pride that motivate him or her to run each day in order to participate in the marathon.

We often have more than one emotion at the same time. I'm excited about my new job, and I'm anxious over whether I can handle it. I'm angry at how you're treating me, and I feel superior because I've never treated you so badly. Here's one I know all too well: The airline lost my luggage, and I'm simultaneously angry over their carelessness, worried because my medicine was in there, embarrassed because I'll have to attend a meeting dressed in what I wore on the plane, and discouraged because I know they'll never find my suitcase before my trip is over.

We can even have emotions about emotions. We call them *meta-emotions*. I could be afraid of public speaking and embarrassed about being afraid. Or I'm being bullied so I feel victimized, and I'm ashamed of myself for allowing that to happen.

A *mood* is more diffuse and less intense than an emotion or a feeling but longer lasting. Most typically, we don't quite know why we're feeling the way we are during a mood, but we are very certain when feeling an emotion. Moods also can be the aftermath of an emotion. Have you ever been annoyed at someone, couldn't stop thinking about it, and ended up in a bad mood? Often, it doesn't feel as though anything caused it—it's just a state of being, but one that's completely tied in with our emotional responses to life. "Mood disorder" is a common term nowadays, describing a psychiatric condition such as depression, bipolarity, or anxiety disorder. These all impair everyday functioning—they're at the extreme of how mood affects our lives.

In addition to emotions, feelings, and moods, there are emotion-related *personality traits*. This feels like who we are, at our core—our predisposition to feel, think, and act in a particular way. We're optimists or pessimists, we're take-charge types or fatalists, we're introverts or extroverts, we're calm or hyper. To be sure, personality traits can change over time, but when they do, it happens gradually. This means we need patience with kids who are growing into themselves. But for the most part, traits are the constants, which can have influence over how we feel but should not be confused with feelings. People who are more optimistic tend to experience greater positive emotions, but they also can overestimate other people's positive emotions.

All of these distinctions matter more to research psychologists and social scientists than to anyone else. For our purposes, we'll use the words *emotions* and *feelings* to mean more or less the same thing. But we'll all better understand our emotional lives if we have the vocabulary to express every nuance of what we feel.

On the road to becoming emotion scientists, we need to avoid the temptation to act as emotion judges.

In both cases, we're attempting to recognize emotions and their source and then to foresee how they might be influencing our thoughts and actions. But an emotion scientist seeks to understand without making value judgments or rendering opinions about whether feelings are justified or not, beneficial or not, or reflecting an objective reality. An emotion scientist comes equipped only with questions and a desire to listen and learn.

An emotion judge, on the other hand, is seeking something else. An emotion judge attempts to evaluate feelings (even his or her own— we're not immune to harsh self-judgment) and deem them good or bad, useful or harmful, grounded in reality or a figment of the imagination. An emotion judge wants the power to validate feelings or negate them—to pass judgment.

Their reasons are understandable. A parent, for instance, has a lot on the line when it comes to a child's emotional life. Any negative feelings that are expressed—anxiety, rage, shame—can be seen as a reflection of the child's upbringing. If an employee feels browbeaten, if a loved one feels despair, if you yourself feel worthless, there's a temptation to deflect responsibility and assign guilt. This is why it's easier to sentence an angry child to a time-out than it is to listen to his or her feelings and explore what's lurking behind them. Where emotion scientists operate with open minds and good intentions, emotion judges are afraid of hearing something dreadful. They come prepared to deny, defend, and blame.

Carol Dweck, a professor at Stanford University and author of the bestselling book *Mindset,* has shown in decades of research how our beliefs about skills determine our success or failure at developing them. Here's what that means: When we believe that emotion skills can be taught, we have greater faith in their ability to change outcomes for the better. If we think that our emotional makeup is more or less fixed and unchangeable, we're less likely to invest much time or effort in developing our own skills or teaching them to others. Emotion scientists share the mindset that says education is possible. To an emotion judge, all that remains is to deem someone's emotional state helpful or harmful, positive or negative, good or bad, without a hope for growth and improvement.

In our judicial system, judges play a valuable and necessary role. In our emotional lives, it's just the opposite.

Having a high degree of emotional intelligence, and possessing what I've described as the five necessary emotion skills, makes all our lives better. Sounds obvious, I realize, but if we need evidence, there's plenty of science to back it up.

The work of researchers Jeremy Yip, an assistant professor at Georgetown University, and Stéphane Côté, a professor at the Rotman School of Management, University of Toronto, demonstrated the concept at the heart of this: Individuals with more developed emotion skills were better able to correctly identify the events that caused their emotions and, therefore, were able to screen out the influence of incidental emotions on their decisions.

We base most of life's decisions on how we think our actions will make us feel. But without emotion skills, research shows that we are notoriously bad at predicting what will make us happy. Many of us have spent time chasing the wrong goals or refusing to engage in activities that actually might make us feel better. We eat sugar to lift a depressed mood when exercise likely will do a better job; we engage with social media to feel connected when we know it amplifies anxiety.

Back when John Kerry ran for president against George W. Bush, we surveyed Yale students to see how angry they would be if their candidate lost. After the election, we tested Kerry voters and found that they had grossly overestimated how mad they would be. In a second study conducted at Duke University, we asked students to predict their feelings about an upcoming basketball game against the school's archrival, University of North Carolina. They were told to imagine how excited they would be if Duke won. They were also asked to predict how they would feel if Duke lost. The day after the game—which UNC won—the students were called and asked to report their levels of excitement. Again, participants overestimated how they would feel. However, in both studies, students who had higher emotional intelligence scores were better at anticipating their emotions. Emotionally intelligent individuals had an intuitive understanding of one of the central conclusions of happiness research: Well-being depends less on objective events than on how those events are perceived, dealt with, and shared with others. Because emotionally skilled people are more likely to recognize this core concept, they are likely to have an advantage in their decision making.

These are critical skills at all ages. Will our children be able to resist the temptation of hurting a friend or alcohol and drug abuse? Will they know how to use their creativity to push beyond boredom and not surrender to it? Will they understand how emotional upsets may lead them to consider poor decisions on social media, then adjust their thinking accordingly? Teaching them emotion skills will help, and there's research to prove it. Young school-age children with more developed emotion skills have fewer conduct problems, are better adjusted, and perform better academically than children with less developed skills.

We're all familiar—firsthand—with the dramatic emotion sensitivities and emotional dysregulations that come with adolescence. They can undermine the success of even the smartest, hardest-working students. But emotional intelligence makes a big difference. The ability of young people to thrive even when feelings (positive *or* negative) threaten to overwhelm their intentions is associated with more developed emotion skills.

Among adolescents, higher emotional intelligence is associated with less depression and anxiety and may be a protective factor against suicidal behavior. Those who are higher in emotional intelligence also are rated both by themselves and by their teachers as being easier to get along with than students with less developed skills. There is also data suggesting that emotional intelligence is related to higher SAT scores, greater creativity, and better grades among high school and college students. In one study, emotional intelligence was a predictor of academic success above grit, a well-known predictor of achievement.

The benefits don't go away once we reach adulthood. Individuals who score higher on emotional intelligence tests tend to report better relationships with friends, parents, and romantic partners. Makes sense. They're more likely to accurately interpret nonverbal cues, understand someone else's feelings, and know which strategies could support another person to feel something more or less.

Research has also linked emotional intelligence to important health and workplace outcomes, including less anxiety, depression, stress, and burnout and greater performance and leadership ability. Individuals with higher emotional intelligence scores also tend to perform better particularly in service-oriented jobs and those involving contact with customers. Think about the reasons you return to the same coffee shop or restaurant. Might it be more about how the barista makes you feel than it is about the coffee or the food?

In two studies, emotion skills correlated with leadership emergence, which is defined as the extent to which someone not in an official position exerts influence over his or her colleagues. Other studies have shown promising associations between emotional intelligence and "transformational" leadership—the kind where leaders motivate and inspire their subordinates to work toward a common vision.

When you have emotion skills, you are perceived by peers to be more sensitive; you have better relationships with colleagues and romantic partners; and you are seen as more confident and secure.

A number of researchers have examined whether emotion skills can be learned in brief interventions. One study found that athletes randomly assigned to participate in ten three-hour workshops had significantly higher emotional intelligence scores post-test than before and had significantly higher scores than their peers in the control group. A second study found similar results among business school students. Participants assigned to a sixteen-hour, not-for-credit course in emotional intelligence showed a significant gain in overall emotional intelligence, while the pre- and post-test scores of their peers in an attention control (that is, business etiquette) course showed no significant change. In our own research we found that classrooms that implemented RULER (the name of our center's systemic, evidence-based approach to social and emotional learning) with the greatest fidelity had students with more developed emotion skills after ten months compared with classrooms that implemented RULER with less fidelity.

Having emotion skills—giving yourself and those around you the permission to feel—doesn't mean you become a doormat or you roll over and agree with everything everyone else says or does. People higher in emotional intelligence are just as likely to push back when attacked— but they will have an easier time dealing with the emotions in a confrontation and will be more skillful at finding a peaceful solution.

None of this means that the emotionally wise person is perfect. You're tired, you're angry, you're worried about something, and so naturally you may not pause to think before you react. You have to give yourself permission to feel even that. You're going to fly off the handle. You're a work in progress. If you mishandled it today, and you have sufficient emotion skills to recognize that, you may do better tomorrow.

It's not always easy to reckon with our own and others' emotional lives. But when kids and adults are given the permission to feel all emotions, and learn how to manage them, it opens doors to collaboration, relationship building, improved decision making and performance, and greater well-being. Almost all the essential ingredients for success arise from emotion skills.

When I give talks, I share the research on emotional intelligence and then ask people about the importance of developing the skills. Naturally, everyone agrees that they are essential. But we keep putting off their acquisition. Students will tell me, *As soon as I get through high school and these tests . . . As soon as I get accepted into graduate school . . .* And then, too soon, they're adults. They are the future doctors, teachers, flight attendants, lawyers, and everyone else who tells us they feel "stressed" most of their waking hours. This isn't how life is supposed to be. But it's how life typically is when we're raised in families, taught in schools, and work in institutions that ignore the importance of emotions.

By failing to address the most significant element of what makes us human, we are choking off the fire of passion and purpose, stunting and distorting the growth and maturity of entire generations, and burning out the adults who are there to help them grow. Emotion skills are the missing link in a child's ability to grow up to be a successful adult. It's up to us to launch the revolution in which the permission to feel drives our success in ways we have yet to imagine.

Again, the necessary skills:

The first step is to recognize what we're feeling.

The second step is to understand what we've discovered—what we're feeling and why.

The next step is to properly label our emotions, meaning not just to call ourselves "happy" or "sad" but to dig deeper and identify the nuances and intricacies of what we feel.

The fourth step is to express our feelings, to ourselves first and then, when right, to others.

The final step is to regulate—as we've said, not to suppress or ignore our emotions but to use them wisely to achieve desired goals.

In the next section, we'll take those steps one by one.

PART TWO

THE RULER SKILLS

4

R: Recognizing Emotion

HERE, AGAIN, IS THE key question: How are you feeling?

This time, before you answer, stop and *don't* think. Just sense it. *Feel* it. It might help to take a slow, deep breath.

My guess is that if you can turn off your analytic mind for a moment, you will get a clear—*visceral*—sense of your underlying emotional state. You know what I'm talking about, even if you don't always put it into words. I mean your basic, fundamental state, right now:

I feel great.

I'm fine.

I feel bleh.

I'm stressed.

You don't even have to use words to articulate it—yet. That will come later. But we can't get there without first being here.

We need to pause—to physically stop whatever we're doing, check in with the state of our minds and bodies, and ask ourselves: At this exact moment, what is my emotional state? Am I feeling up or down? Pleasant or unpleasant? Would I like to approach the world or steer clear? Next, let's check for physical clues. Am I energized or depleted? Is my heart racing, am I clenching my fists, is there a knot in my stomach, or am I feeling balanced, cool, and at ease?

The first of the RULER skills we need to acquire in order to become emotion scientists is Recognition. That's what we're learning in this chapter: simply how to recognize emotions in ourselves and others with accuracy.

As we've seen, asking people to find the words for what they're feeling doesn't always produce the desired result. Over the past decade, I've asked hundreds of thousands of adults—from educators to parents to physicians to CEOs—why it's so hard for them to describe how they're feeling. This is what I hear:

"We never stop to ask ourselves that question."

"We were never taught a comprehensive emotion vocabulary."

"We're used to saying fine or okay, automatically."

"It's not always safe to share how you really feel."

"Nobody actually *cares* how you feel."

"We've been taught to not discuss our feelings."

"If we acknowledge how we feel, we'll have to own it and *do* something about it."

"Emotions are unnatural."

"I don't want to be judged."

"There's no time!"

"I have ten feelings."

"There is too much social pressure to risk being honest."

"If I shared how I felt, no one would want to be around me."

"I feel as if I grew up in the witness protection program. We were told to never share anything."

You can see what we're up against. But until we can recognize our own emotions, we can't learn the skills necessary for regulating them. To recognize our emotions is to acknowledge that we're all feeling beings and we're experiencing emotions every instant of our lives.

And Recognition doesn't apply only to our own feelings—we need to be able to recognize them in other people too. That's a bit more challenging because you can't constantly ask someone, "Hi, what's your basic, underlying emotional state right now?" (Trust me, try it once and see.) But unless we're mind readers, we can go only by appearances, which are not always accurate indicators, or by our intuition, which works best with people we know well but not with the rest of the world.

Recognition is especially critical because most of our communication is nonverbal. This includes everything from facial expressions to body language to vocal tones—not the words but simply the way we say them. Words can lie or hide the truth. Physical gestures rarely do. That underscores the importance of the first R in RULER—it requires us to recognize a person's general emotion or mood before attempting to get at the details of exactly what he or she is feeling and why. It points us in the right direction.

Here's what can happen when we don't recognize something as basic as another person's emotional state. An engaged, friendly child becomes increasingly hostile. A teenager who was once bright and bubbly becomes lethargic and barely functional. An adult who used to radiate well-being now suffers from crippling anxiety. And in the worst-case scenarios, people become mysteriously depressed and are now gone, by their own hand. After the fact, we often find the same thing: a bullied, abused, or alienated adult or child who was ignored but would have benefited from outside intervention. We look at one another and ask, "How did everybody miss the signals?" As a child, I was secure in the knowledge that I was loved by my parents. However, I went to school every day and played after school on our street where I was being abused and bullied for many years. How did this go unnoticed? All the obvious signs were there. But loving me was not synonymous with *seeing* me.

There are times when we express our negative feelings in behavior that is itself destructive, off-putting, unbearable. At moments like these, we practically defy the people in our lives to reach out and engage with us or try to help. Other times we alienate ourselves, avoid being with friends, and withdraw from social activities. At these moments, we send signals that we just want to be alone or that everything is okay, when it's not. In my childhood, I was a textbook example of self-defeating outbursts and calculated seclusion. But these are the times when we need to try hardest to break through the displays of rage or self-alienation. This is when we must remember that our behavior sometimes sends the exact opposite message of what we really need. Our actions scream, "Get away!" or, "I'm fine!" while our emotions beg for attention.

The first step toward fully engaging with our own and someone else's emotions—even before we know the specifics of what's causing those feelings—is developing the skill of Recognition.

There's a tool that can help.

The Mood Meter was built based on what is called "the circumplex model of emotion," as developed by James Russell, a professor at Boston College. He said that human emotions have two core properties or dimensions—energy and pleasantness. Russell had the insight to intersect these dimensions to create a single graph that could represent all feelings. The horizontal axis represents the degree of pleasantness, from very unpleasant to very pleasant. The vertical axis represents the degree of energy, from very low to very high.

Those two forces alone tell us a great deal about our emotional lives at any given moment. Even when we are not aware of how we are feeling, our emotion system is continuously monitoring our surroundings for changes that may be relevant to our goals, values, and well-being.

As a tool to help people recognize emotions, the Mood Meter was first used in *The Emotionally Intelligent Manager,* a 2004 book by David Caruso and Peter Salovey. Later, Caruso and I built on that and developed it into the centerpiece of RULER, our evidence-based approach to social and emotional learning that currently is in more than two thousand schools and districts in the United States and in other countries, including Australia, China, England, Italy, Mexico, and Spain.

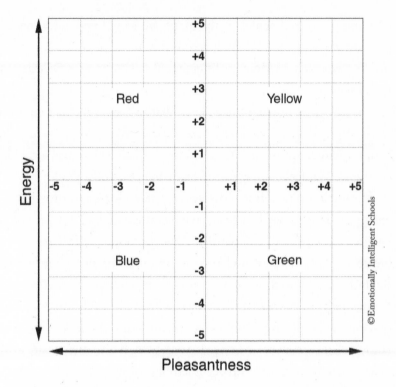

The Mood Meter is designed to chart every feeling a human being can experience and project it onto a graph similar to the one Russell proposed. It allows us to chart our observations about pleasantness and energy in order to understand key information about emotions at a glance. Using the tool, we can readily visualize hundreds of emotions, from rage to serenity, ecstasy to despair, their co-occurrences, and everything in between.

As you can see in the figure above (and on the endpapers), the Mood Meter is a square divided evenly by the horizontal axis (pleasantness) and vertical axis (energy) into four quadrants. At the far left end of the horizontal axis is the extreme of unpleasantness, which we represent with a –5; at the far right end is its opposite—very pleasant, at +5. Likewise, at the top of the vertical axis is high energy and at the bottom is the opposite. We measure everything on both axes by a number—at dead center of the graph we would be neutral on both pleasantness and energy, which is scored as 0.

We gave each quadrant a different color, chosen to reflect its emotional state.

The top right quadrant is yellow. That's where we experience high levels of pleasantness *and* energy. If you're in the yellow, you're feeling happy, excited, optimistic. Your posture is likely erect, your eyes likely sparkling. You feel energized and ready to take on the world.

The top left is red. This is the quadrant for low pleasantness but high energy. Here you may be angry, anxious, frustrated, or scared, but also passionate, assertive, competitive. Your body might feel tense, your breath is likely shallow, and your heart might be pumping fast. You might have furrowed or raised eyebrows depending on whether you're feeling angry or afraid. You're preparing to fight or flee; maybe you're psyching yourself up to win a race; or you might be preparing to valiantly defend someone who needs your help. No matter what, in this quadrant, you are in the grip of something strong.

The bottom right is green, for high pleasantness but low energy. Here you're peaceful, contented, serene—and mellow. Your body likely feels at ease, you're breathing slowly. You have a gentle smile and feel safe and secure.

And the bottom left is blue, indicating low pleasantness *and* energy— which could be anything from sadness to apathy to outright depression, but also empathy and concern. Your gaze might be down, you might have a frown on your face, and your body posture likely is slumped. You feel like retreating or disappearing or have the desire to comfort someone who has experienced a misfortune.

In the coming chapters, we'll get into the intricacies of the Mood Meter as we discuss each emotion and its exact position. For now, we'll concern ourselves with the four quadrants only.

Maybe a few examples will help.

It's a Saturday morning in spring, the weather is gorgeous, and I'm sitting in a garden surrounded by flowers and budding trees. Okay, you don't need a PhD to know that I'm pretty high on the pleasant-ness scale—deep into the green quadrant if it's a sleepy Saturday morning. If I were just as happy but feeling supercharged, I'd be up in the yellow.

Or, I arrive at the airport for a work trip, and as I'm checking in I sud-denly realize I don't have my laptop. Did I leave it at home? Did I leave it in the car? No time to go back and find it. Right now, I'm at the highest intensity for sure and also in the quadrant of extreme unpleasantness—deep in the red zone. Once I glumly accept that it's a lost cause and I'm probably not going to have the laptop for my presentation, I may slip over into the blue—low on pleasantness *and* energy.

Recognition is the key first step toward understanding anyone's—our own or someone else's—present emotional state. Unfortunately, it's not foolproof. There are many ways to misunderstand what's right before our eyes and ears. This is why the four other skills that we'll discuss in the following chapters are so important.

A few stories to explain what I mean:

I have a relative who never has a nice word for anyone. (I have to be careful here—I don't want to make him too recognizable!) He's the most negative person I've ever known, with a huge chip on his shoul-der. If he weren't family, none of us would put up with him.

It's my habit at family gatherings to bring along facial expression recognition materials that research psychologists use in experiments. These are photos of people displaying typical emotions, scientifically designed to be as universal as possible. You're supposed to look at the face and identify what the person is feeling. I make it into a kind of parlor game, but I always learn something along the way.

I showed my relative a photo of a person expressing fear.

"All right," I said, "tell me what you think she's feeling."

"Looks like anger to me," he said.

"But do you see how her eyes are wide open?" I asked him. "And her mouth is slightly open and turned down? Doesn't that look more like fear, or even like angst?"

"Maybe it's fear to you," he said, "but it's anger to me." Which made perfect sense—through his eyes, *everything* looks like anger.

Once, at a dinner with friends and colleagues, I tried something else I'll do from time to time at gatherings. I went around the table and asked people where they believe they live, emotionally speaking.

"I think I'm kind of bubbly and happy," one woman said.

"Really?" another friend replied. "I'm surprised to hear that. I don't see you that way at all."

I moved on to someone else, who said he feels as though he comes across as calm and relaxed.

"Well, *I* always thought you were kind of anxious," the same friend told him.

It went on that way for a while.

After dinner, I took this friend aside and pointed out that in every case, she shared a more negative view of people than they had of themselves. She was mortified and shocked—it didn't occur to her that her view of anyone was particularly sour. But it surely was.

A final story, one that took place when I was still a graduate student. A friend had just experienced something truly disturbing, and she was telling me all about it, weeping as she spoke. Just then, another student—one who was notoriously self-involved—came breezing by, stopped, and said, "You'll never believe what my boyfriend and I did over the weekend!"

My friend and I looked up, stunned. We had never seen somebody misread all the cues so badly.

Sometimes even I am prone to misinterpretation, even though I've devoted significant time to studying this. I had a graduate student who developed a strange habit—when she had to turn in a paper, she would come into my office, toss it on my desk, and then run out without saying a word.

Finally, I asked her about this, and she told me that when I was reading her work a look of disgust would come over my face. She couldn't bear watching, she said, which was why she would flee. I was shocked—I had absolutely no problem with her work. Part of this student's reaction may have been her own insecurity about her writing. But the truth is that I have no idea what signals I may have been sending while I was concentrating on grading papers. Either way, she was responding to something, and it was getting in the way of our working relationship.

We've all sometimes misunderstood other people's emotions when we based our assumptions only on unspoken signals. But often, that's the only evidence we have.

In my work, I come up against this all the time. When I conduct seminars for educators, I'll often ask the room how skilled they are at recognizing students' emotions. Everyone says, "Well, this is what we do all day, every day."

"Great," I say. "I'm going to express an emotion, and all of you will write down what feeling you detect." Then I turn my back on the room, assume a facial expression, and turn around again.

"Okay," I'll ask after a few moments, "what do you think I was feeling?"

One person will say I was angry. Another says I looked calm. To a third, I seemed disapproving. One thinks I was flirting with her. Someone else says she couldn't tell what I was feeling.

Actually, I tell them, I was trying to express contentment. That leads to the discussion of who (if anyone) was right. I know what I was trying to display, but does that mean I know how I was coming across? Observers are often certain they know how I feel. I recall one participant who said, "Marc, I don't think you're even aware of what you were really displaying." It's possible I'm no more of an expert on my own emotional expressions than anyone else. But the fact is that we are making these automatic judgments about how people feel all day long—and we're often wrong. Think about the implications. How often are you misread? How often are you misreading those around you? Do you even know?

Of course, if I display a very conspicuous emotion, such as surprise—eyes popped open wide, mouth agape—everyone gets it right. But how often do we get surprised in a day?

Given all that, it's easy to see why emotion science must rely so heavily on verbal communication—knowing which questions to ask other people and how to listen and process the answers. We also have to articulate what we're feeling, especially the subtleties that distinguish one emotion from another that's close but not quite the same. Otherwise we'll never reach our ultimate goal: understanding, communicating, and regulating our emotions effectively so that they become a help and not a hindrance.

"The human face—in repose and in movement, at the moment of death as in life, in silence and in speech, when seen or sensed from within, in actuality or as represented in art or recorded by the camera—is a commanding, complicated, and at times confusing source of information," rhapsodized Paul Ekman, the legendary psychologist who is known as the greatest human lie detector and was the inspiration for the TV series *Lie to Me*.

Imagine trying to keep track of every possible facial expression of emotion! Many of those are so-called microexpressions, the kind that briefly flicker across one's features, so quickly they're barely visible. Could any of us, even Dr. Ekman, track so much emotional activity day in and day out?

Still, we have all spent our entire lives, from before we can remember, studying facial expressions for their emotional content. It's the basis for all human relationships, starting with mother and newborn. We do it instinctively, as a matter of survival, because the better we are at reading facial expressions, the more we'll know about the intentions of the people around us. We've all evolved to become emotion scientists. But we still need to learn the skills.

A century before Ekman, in 1872, Charles Darwin published his third major work, *The Expression of the Emotions in Man and Animals*. In it, he wrote that animals and humans both express their emotions physically, and there are some universals of expression among people—raised eyebrows denoting surprise, for example—as well as great diversity in emotion expression.

Ekman and other psychologists ran a series of cross-cultural studies in the 1970s, making the case that all human faces express six "basic emotions" in much the same way:

Happiness
Sadness
Anger
Fear
Surprise
Disgust

Sounds about right. But then the literature goes on to say that we all display these emotions in more or less the same fashion, and that's where it gets a little murky. We academics all make ample use of those materials depicting prototypical facial expressions of different emotions that I bring to family gatherings. But we know it's a stretch to say that everybody everywhere manifests these emotions in exactly the same way.

Certainly there's something universal about those six. From childhood on, we're all capable of making the faces associated with those emotions. We don't require lessons—we inherently understand them. More recent research by Dacher Keltner, a professor at the University of California–Berkeley, and his colleagues suggests that as many as twenty-two emotions are recognized in the face at above-chance levels (that is, above 50/50) across different cultures.

We also rely on sound for hints of someone's emotional state. Tone of voice can send an unmistakable message—when we're angry or sad or frightened, we may sound alike no matter what language we speak. In one study, college students from ten different countries and villagers in

remote Bhutan were all tested to see if they could match the spontaneous sounds we make when inspired by various emotions—amusement,
awe, contempt, relief, sympathy, triumph, sixteen in all—with stories
that elicited the same feeling. They found "very strong recognition" in
all eleven cultures. In another study, subjects were extremely proficient
at distinguishing fake laughter from real.

In a series of clever studies, researchers showed that emotions also
can be detected in touch. Two participants, one assigned to be the encoder and the other the decoder, were asked to work together. The decoder was instructed to sit at a table separated by a curtain. The encoder
was given a list of emotions and asked to communicate thirteen different ones on the decoder's arm, using any form of touch that lasted
a second or two. Of the so-called basic or universal emotions, anger,
fear, and disgust were reliably decoded. Pro-social emotions, those that
help us build and maintain relationships, such as love, gratitude, and
sympathy, also were easily detected. Self-focused emotions such as embarrassment, pride, and envy were not detected, as might be predicted.
Given their communicative function, it makes sense that we are better
able to recognize social emotions than self-focused ones through touch.

As we discussed earlier, the primary emotional message we interpret from reading people's emotions, strangers or intimates alike, is to
either approach or avoid—or freeze to some extent, as with surprise.
We welcome people into our circle, or we warn them to keep their
distance. If I'm a teacher or a parent, the approach-or-avoid dynamic is
what tells our children whether they are valued or dismissed, loved or
just tolerated. We send the same signals to our fellow adults too.

Accurately reading nonverbal cues—facial expressions, vocal tones,
body language—makes social interaction possible. It tells us how (or
even if) to start a conversation, whether a person is paying attention or
not, if we're dealing with someone we'd rather avoid or who truly needs
to engage with us right now. An expression as simple as a smile can signify emotions and intentions ranging from joy, interest, and romantic
attraction to disapproval, deference, and even aggression. Interestingly,

a sincere smile tends to last for a few seconds, whereas a polite or disingenuous smile tends to last for just a quarter second.

Psychologists are fond of testing how we register and analyze the nonverbal cues of emotion. They typically show subjects photos of faces displaying all the usual expressions—smiling, frowning, eyes popped wide open or narrowed, lips parted and teeth showing or mouths clamped shut. But the cues are fairly obvious—there's a big difference in my face if I just hit the lottery or broke my toe. If I show you a face with furrowed eyebrows, piercing eyes, and pressed lips, you don't have to be a genius to see anger. Still, they don't reflect real life—how often do we see full-blown anger in a business meeting? In real time, the emotions we're attempting to read in others are a good deal more subtle, ambiguous, fleeting, and mixed.

However, for all those universals in reading emotional states, there are complex differences, too, depending on a variety of factors.

Cultural influences matter. We are more accurate at reading emotions of people from our own cultural background. In addition, people from different cultures tend to attribute varied meanings to facial expressions. In one study, Japanese and American participants were shown images of people displaying a happy expression. The Japanese rated the person's inner experience and outward expression at the same level of happiness. The Americans thought that the external display was more intense than the person's actual inner experience.

There are also differences due to personality. People who are agreeable, one of the "big five" personality traits, tend to perceive people who are displaying angry or hostile facial expressions as being friendlier than they really are. There are even differences based on relationship quality. A colleague I've worked with for fifteen years is reliably better than anyone else at identifying when I am bored. Finally, there are differences based on context or setting. Our interpretation of someone's gritted teeth and clenched fist will be different if they are at a political rally or in a brawl at a bar. In one study, people's ratings of a facial expression meant to depict disgust ranged from 91 percent when a person was holding a soiled article to only 11 percent when the person had clenched fists. In the real world, all those neat categories of emotion no longer work so well at interpreting others' inner lives.

Our perception of emotion is easily swayed by the opinions of others. In a classic study, a person posing as a visiting professor gave a lecture to university students. Before the speaker appeared, half of the students received information that he was a rather warm person. The other half of the students were told that he was cold. The second group of students perceived the lecturer to be more irritable than those who were told he was a nice guy.

There are also other prejudices—gender stereotypes and racial implicit bias (both attitudes that affect our actions and decisions in an unconscious manner)—that influence how we read emotions. We are more likely to detect anger in men's expressions of emotion but sadness in women's. U.S. participants are more likely to perceive anger in the emotional expressions of African Americans. Chinese participants' scores on a pro-Chinese/anti-white implicit bias test correlate with their ratings of the intensity of white subjects' angry, fearful, and sad facial expressions.

No wonder we're all so prone to being misinterpreted and to misunderstanding the emotional states of others. We make fatal miscalculations—judging by his stone-faced expression when I said hello to my boss this morning, he's clearly disappointed with the report I turned in yesterday. How was I to know that he had just come from a tough meeting with *his* boss? The term psychologists use for this phenomenon is "attribution bias," meaning we observe someone's cues or behavior and wrongly attribute them to our own emotional state.

We saw how my relative responded to the photo I showed him. His own emotional state overpowered his ability to objectively look at someone else and see what they feel. In my relative's case there's an even more precise term: "hostile attribution bias," since his own anger causes him to see that same emotion everywhere, even where it may not exist. Back in the eighteenth century, the poet Alexander Pope said it well: "All looks yellow to the jaundiced eye." If you go through life angry, you will see anger everywhere you look. The same is true of other emotions—even positive ones.

It's human nature to pay more attention to negative emotional information than positive. Starting in childhood, it's how we rely on the reactions of other people to measure the danger in any given situation. This is the reason kids study their parents' faces before trying anything potentially risky—they're searching for a clue as to how risky it might really be.

Still, some of us are more prone than others to sensing negative emotions. When looking at faces with neutral expressions, depressed people are more likely to read them as sad than happy; those with anxiety disorders tend to see fear; people who grew up in homes where parents argued frequently see anger; irritable children see hostility or fear. Brain scientists have even identified where in the brain this bias might reside—in the perigenual anterior cingulate cortex (the pgACC for short).

Here's a question I get often: Are we actually getting worse at reading one another's emotions? There's evidence that says we are. The more time we spend communicating through electronic screens, the less face-to-face (or even voice-to-ear) time we spend and the less practice we get at reading the nonverbal cues. In one study, sixth graders who went five days without glancing at a smartphone or other digital screen were better at reading emotions than their peers from the same school who continued to spend hours each day looking at their phones, tablets, computers, and so on.

And that's not the only obstacle modern life poses. At a seminar I taught in Los Angeles, a principal stood up and said she was concerned that students today could have extra difficulty decoding facial expressions owing to the popularity—especially in her hometown—of Botox. Which makes perfect sense, because how could you tell how Mom and Dad feel if their foreheads, eyebrows, and corners of their eyes and mouths have been chemically paralyzed?

. . .

The recognition skill improves only with practice. And because it relies on nonverbal information, we have to be sensitive to the sensations and nuances of emotions, our own and those of other people. If you over-think it, you're doing it wrong. At this point in the process, we're not looking to nail down the precise emotion, just the general area where it exists—the quadrant of the Mood Meter. Are we feeling up or down? Pleasant or unpleasant? It's the kind of question you can ask yourself every hour on the hour and get a different answer. You can try the same thing with the people in your life—whether it's your spouse, your boss, your kids, or the desk clerk at the library. There's no penalty for explor-ing and quite a bit of potential benefit from developing this skill. In any event, it's the first necessary step.

However, as we've seen, we can't rely solely on that visceral sense to tell us everything we need to know. For that, we must go deeper. We also have to allow for the possibility that we can be wrong. As we've seen, there are many ways to misunderstand and misinterpret non-verbal communication. It's okay to misidentify once in a while. That's what the following steps are for—to correct our paths and bring us closer to understanding. Because in order to know an emotion, our own or someone else's, we need to know what's behind it—its causes. For that, we need the U—as in Understanding emotion.

5

U: Understanding Emotion

Let's start this chapter with a slightly different question: How am *I* feeling?

Or, more precisely, how *was* I feeling?

When I was thirteen, and the victim of daily bullying in school, my dad pushed me to do martial arts—to toughen me up. He was a strong guy from the Bronx and only ever wanted the same for me. (Now, I've had a fifth-degree black belt in Hapkido, a Korean martial art, for a long time and it still has not made me a tough guy.)

I wasn't even athletic back then, but I was determined to make my dad happy, so I tried. Before long, I was gearing up to qualify for my yellow belt. I practiced every day for three months and then literally begged my martial arts instructor to let me take the test early.

The big day finally came. I had to perform a series of kicks, punches, blocks, and self-defense moves. I was so nervous I didn't even want my mom in the studio, so she waited in the car.

And then I failed the test.

I left the studio, opened the car door, got in, and started screaming,

"I hate you! I'm never going back to Hapkido again! I'm a loser! You should never have let me go! You knew I'd never be good at it! And I'm not going to school tomorrow either!" Total freak-out.

Okay, how am I feeling?

When I role-play this story during presentations and ask people what they think, their most common answers are anger, disappointment, embarrassment, humiliation. Certainly those are all fair assumptions based on my behavior, but really, they're just guessing. All my listeners have to go on is their intuition and my howls of hurt. They're committing one of a couple of possible attribution biases: either they're inferring how I'm feeling based solely on my behavior—or they're labeling my emotions based on how they believe *they'd* feel in that situation. We can't really call these people emotion scientists at this point. They don't know enough to say what I was feeling or why, and they haven't done anything to find out. We adults want to believe that the emotional lives of children are less complex and messy than our own, but it's not so. Indeed, sometimes the opposite is true.

Now, put yourself in my mother's place. She's in the car, waiting, praying that I'll pass the test for the sake of my self-esteem if nothing else. She's watching the studio door, trying to read my body language as I emerge.

And then she gets an earful. If she had any intention of finding out why I was overcome by so many horrible emotions, that good impulse was drowned out by my fury. My outrage triggered hers, and she yelled right back, "Stop screaming at me! How dare you talk to me this way! Stop it this instant! Wait until I tell your father how you're treating me!"

Not exactly what I needed at that moment. But it's what I was accustomed to getting from my parents. It's not that they didn't want to do better. They just had no idea how. The way they treated me was probably the way they were treated when they were children. Pain isn't pretty. And so the refusal to acknowledge unhappy childhood emotion, or the inability to deal with it, gets handed down from one generation to the next.

What exactly was needed at that moment? Well, you could say "understanding" and you'd be right. But what exactly are we trying to understand? And how do we go about it?

Of all the five RULER skills required to be an emotion scientist, this is one of the most challenging to acquire. In the previous chapter, we learned about the importance of being able to discern our own feelings and to read, at a glance or soon thereafter, someone else's overall emotional state. And with that, we took the important first step toward emotional well-being.

Now, the real work begins.

Here is where we have to decide whether we even wish to understand what might have caused our own or the other person's feelings. This is certainly true of our own feelings—there are plenty of times when it's easiest to take whatever emotion we're experiencing and hide it in an airtight compartment, to be dealt with at a more convenient time (maybe). This is also the moment of truth when we're faced with exploring someone else's feelings. It's like opening Pandora's box: we don't know what will emerge, or how it will affect us, or—most critically—what we'll be expected to do about it.

All this drama is triggered by a single word: *Why?* Why this feeling? Why now? Understanding emotions begins when we start to answer that question—why do you or I feel this way? What is the underlying reason for this feeling? What's causing it? It's rarely a simple matter. There may be a complex web of events and memories, of one emotion provoking another. Usually, asking one question will lead to more questions, a succession of follow-ups that can go deep. Like peeling the layers of an onion. No wonder it's scary: once we start asking, there's no turning back.

Understanding emotions is a journey. Possibly an adventure. When it's finished, we may find ourselves someplace new, someplace unexpected, somewhere, perhaps, we had no intention of going. And yet there we are, wiser than before—maybe wiser than we wished to be. But there's no other way forward.

If we're faced with the emotions of someone close to us—a loved one, a valued colleague, a good friend—the stakes are even higher, because now there's a distinct possibility that we are somehow complicit. That something we've said or done (or failed to do) is the reason for the difficult feelings that confront us. Here's where we take a deep breath before we start digging. This, I can imagine now, is how my parents must have felt during the worst days of my childhood: *What if this is our fault?*

The core skill of Understanding is the search for the underlying *theme* or possible cause that fuels the emotion. We're not asking questions and listening to answers just to provide a sympathetic ear. As we listen, we're looking for a meaning that goes deeper than the words being said.

"I hate school and I'm never going back!" That's important information, but only if we know what to do with it. What's the cause? Is this child afraid of something related to school? Possibly. There are times we hate what we fear. What causes fear? Its underlying theme is danger, threat. So perhaps in this instance hate equals danger, in which case we know the direction our next questions should take.

Now when we ask, "What's happening at school that makes you hate it so much?" we know what to listen for: a potential source of danger. A difficult teacher? An impending bad report card? A schoolyard bully? We suspect it's there somewhere, and we gently investigate until we find it. This is how a scientist operates—with a theory that will be either proved or disproved by further investigation. Maybe it's not fear that's fueling the emotion. Perhaps it's disappointment, or shame. In every case, there's one or a couple of needs or emotional states underlying our feelings, and that's what Understanding helps us to find.

We also need to keep in mind what psychologists refer to as "appraisal theory." Many emotions—both positive and negative—have universal, underlying themes, but their individual causes vary from person to person. All day, each of us rapidly, and even unconsciously, evaluates situations or experiences, and these evaluations lead to different emotions. But what makes me feel excited about public speaking might make you feel terrified. What strikes fear or anxiety into the heart of one person may scarcely register in another. But what matters is the person's experience—that's what we're trying to identify, so we can address it. That's another part of the emotion scientist's skill set—the ability to put aside one's own appraisals so we can comprehend and empathize with those of other people.

Acquiring the Understanding skill is not always such an easy process. Typically, the need to understand an emotion increases with its intensity—the stronger the feeling, the higher the stakes. This is true for us all but especially for children, who don't have the vocabulary, prefrontal cortical circuitry, or presence of mind to make their innermost feelings clear. When a child says, "I hate you!"—as most probably do, sooner or later—we recoil. There are few things more dispiriting a parent can hear. But *hate* in all likelihood isn't really the issue. Those words are fueled by something impossible (in the moment) to articulate. It's the listener's job to remain calm and try to hear the words that aren't being said—yet.

Now, with all that in mind, let's go back to the four quadrants of the Mood Meter and start there. Within each quadrant, there exists a wide range of individual emotions. Knowing these can help us direct our questions.

Yellow, as we've said, is where the high-pleasantness, high-energy feelings are located. These are the emotions of joy, surprise, and excitement, among many others. What's causing them? Something positive and possibly unexpected has happened and we're celebrating inside. We've made significant steps toward an important goal. We're anticipating an event or an experience that will make us happy.

The red quadrant denotes unpleasant emotions that are high in energy. It's red for a reason: this is where anger, fear, and anxiety all are situated. Because these are in some ways similar, it's easy to confuse them. That's a mistake when we're trying to determine what feelings are dictating someone's actions. Red also is where passion lives. Emotions in this quadrant generally make us hyperalert, owing to our perception of opposition. It's the fight-or-flight response that raises our heart rate, respiration, and blood pressure. When angry, we're focused on someone or something external treating us unfairly, unjustly—our attention is pointing outward, hypervigilant, assertive. When fearful, we're alert to impending danger. When we're passionate, our desire is to convince others that our views are correct.

Blue is the space where pleasantness and energy are both low, meaning we might be somewhere on the sadness-depression continuum. Our thinking is narrowly focused and pessimistic. We're looking inward and focused on failure, loss, or whatever else might be causing these feelings.

Green is the space where our pleasantness is high and energy is low. It's the place on the Mood Meter where we generally feel calm or content. Our body and mind are at ease and we feel complete. Our thoughts are focused on ways to appreciate the present moment. Our need to solve problems or fix things is at a minimum.

Now that we know our quadrant, our emotional space, we're ready to zero in on specifics.

These are some of the questions we can ask when we're trying to understand our own feelings:

- What just happened? What was I doing before this happened?
- What might have caused my feelings or reaction?
- What happened this morning, or last night, that might be involved in this?
- What has happened before with this person that might be connected? (In the event that your emotion has to do with a relationship.)
- What memories do I have about this situation or place?

When we're acting as an emotion scientist with someone else, we can ask the other person:

- What might have happened to cause this feeling?
- What usually makes you feel this way?
- What's going on that you're feeling this way?
- What were you doing just before you started feeling this way? Who were you with?
- What do you need right now? What can I do to support you?

As a teaching exercise, we'll sometimes have children read a story, then ask them:

- What does this character feel?
- Why does he or she feel that way? What do you think might have caused this character to feel this way?
- What about what happened to the character helps you to understand his or her feelings?
- If the same thing happened to you, what do you think you would feel?

We can better understand emotions and their linked causes and ramifications by considering them in pairs and groupings. We can develop pattern recognition to help us know what questions to ask as we search for the truth. For example:

Shame, guilt, and embarrassment

Shame is a judgment, but from the outside—from our perception that other people believe we broke a moral or ethical rule or some shared convention. We believe we are diminished in their eyes. A great deal of bullying's damage to the victim, and resulting isolation, comes from this more than any physical suffering.

Guilt is a judgment we make of ourselves when we feel remorse or responsibility for something we did, usually something that feels wrong.

Embarrassment is when we've been caught violating some social norm, such as how to dress for an occasion, or which fork to use, or how to behave in a certain situation. We all have had plenty of such moments and go far out of our way to avoid them.

These three all seem closely related in our emotional lives, but researchers have found that they have unique psychological causes and cognitive-behavioral consequences, which should remind us to distinguish among them when we're searching for the reasons we feel them.

Jealousy and envy

Often, we use the words *jealousy* and *envy* to mean the same thing, but they're different emotions. Jealousy is a form of fear—fear of losing someone important to you, especially to someone else. We've all witnessed (and sometimes even experienced) romantic or sexual jealousy that is coupled with anger or even rage. It's a combustible combination. Children can be jealous of a sibling or classmate when they perceive their parent or teacher spending more time with the other child. They are jealous because they feel threatened and fear the loss of their relationship with the adult or that they're being cheated out of valuable relationship time.

Envy, on the other hand, has to do with wanting something that someone else has. Again, it could be a person or a thing, a position, even a reputation. Envy is caused by our coveting something that's not ours. Envy could lead us to focus our efforts and work harder to attain something desired. In that case, it may be a force for good. But it can also be the opposite—it can lead to resentment and even to aggression toward the person who has what we desire.

Joy and contentment

In most dictionaries the definitions of joy and contentment are nearly identical—"states of being happy and satisfied." But are they *really* the same? On the Mood Meter, we tend to place joy in the yellow quadrant—high pleasantness and energy—whereas contentment is in the green quadrant—high pleasantness but low energy. We do this for a reason: both the subjective experience and core appraisals that cause these emotions are different. Joy *feels* energetic and contentment *feels* calm, and joy is *caused by* a sense of getting what one wants and contentment is *caused by* a sense of completeness (not wanting or needing anything).

For most of us in the West, joy is something we strive for (think the pursuit of happiness). Contentment, however, is more a state of psychological balance, not something we actively pursue—we feel contentment when we cherish the present moment. Research has highlighted the ways in which *happiness* facilitates creativity and social bonds. But what kind of happiness are we referring to? Paradoxical to what we've been taught, the constant pursuit of happiness can be self-defeating. Accumulating research shows that the more we value happiness, the more likely we are to feel disappointed. Thus, although happiness is often seen as highly desirable, we need to distinguish between the different kinds of happiness. Not all of its forms are beneficial for all purposes in life and in every situation.

Stress and pressure

Stress can be deceptive because it's become such a catchall term for children and adults alike. An interlude I had with a student is a perfect example. Here's an email (removing all identifying information) she sent me at nine P.M. on a Sunday before the midterm exam:

> Hey professor!
>
>   I don't know you well enough to know how you feel about these kinds of things, but I was wondering if I could take a makeup exam without a dean's excuse. I was playing in a tournament all weekend, waking up at 6:30 every morning (if you want verification you can go to the website) and I thought I could study each evening

but my parents came with my sister and I've gone out to eat with them and had a banquet with the team one night. Anyway, now I can start studying but I'm *so fucking tired and stressed* and I would like to sleep but I have the exam tomorrow. I understand if you say no, please let me know *asap* however so I know if I can sleep right now or not.

Entitlement and disrespect are triggers for me. So I did what any good professor would do: I didn't respond. Better that than writing something I'd later regret. Truth is, I did reply, but not until after the exam the following day.

She didn't show up for the exam.

When she returned to class, I approached her and said, "I'm not sure about that email. . . ."

She said, "But you're such a fun professor!"

I said, "Fun is one thing, but your email was really *off.*"

A week later, she came to me and said, "I've really thought a lot about what happened, and want to apologize."

I thanked her.

"And I'd really like to work for you," she said.

Surprised, I asked her, "What are you interested in?"

"I'm not really sure," she said, "but when I decide what I'd like to do in your center, I'll let you know."

Again, I was triggered. Who *is* this entitled . . . ?

In that moment, I decided to make her my emotional intelligence project. I asked her to come see me during office hours.

Once there, I said, "First you sent that email about not taking the exam. Then you gave me an attitude in class. Then you said you'd *let me know* what you're interested in when you figure it out. Tell me something: What's going on?"

She said she was under "tremendous stress." Like every other college student, I thought.

"What's *really* going on?" I asked.

She told me that her grandmother had just passed away, that her mother has a fear of dying, that her mother texts her ten times per day and wants her to go home every weekend, or she wants to come to campus to visit her.

That sounded like something more than typical college student stress.

Stress is a response to too many demands and not enough resources—managing both family/work responsibilities and financial burdens—to meet them. Pressure is a situation in which you perceive that something at stake is dependent on the outcome of your performance like performing in front of a group or acing an interview.

In the end, my student really needed support dealing with the *pressure* her mother was putting on her. She had misattributed that pressure as stress about other stuff, such as sports, school, my exam, and so on. It was easier to blame those things than to address the real source of emotional tension in her life—her parent.

But I wouldn't have learned any of that had I been turned off by her attitude, which came across as pure arrogance. I had to probe and keep probing. The questions we ask to understand someone's feelings are necessary to encourage answers that go beyond a simple yes or no, or "I feel angry," or "I feel sad," and so on. We're emotion scientists, remember. We're trying to uncover the deepest of feelings.

But we're not just verbalizing questions—we're also sending unspoken messages as we make our inquiries. I'm talking about the nonverbal cues we display, the facial expressions, body language, and vocal tone that say we're genuinely interested in the answers, that we care about the feelings of the person to whom we're talking and are willing to give this conversation the time and attention it deserves. If I ask about your feelings but I'm glancing at my phone or at the clock on the wall, or if I'm leaning away from you with my arms crossed and my eyes narrowed, the message is clear: I don't really want to know. I'm just waiting for you to say something—*anything*—so I can cut this talk short and do something else.

I may even be sending *this* destructive message: I already know what you're going to say, and I definitely am going to push back. That's not the attitude of an emotion scientist. It's how an emotion judge approaches the situation: just waiting to hear enough to blame you for your feelings and shut this conversation down.

You may remember the story I told earlier about my uncle Marvin and how he got me to open up. He didn't have any trick questions or techniques. His sincere interest in me and how I felt and his obvious desire to help me were all it took. It's impossible to fake.

Understanding is where the science of emotion really becomes a pursuit—almost a detective story. If my mother or father had asked me that day of my Hapkido test, "Marc, what's wrong?" I guarantee that my reply would have been something like "I hate you! Leave me alone!"

An unmistakable expression of rage, but not much else useful there. Clearly, I was expressing an inability or unwillingness to discuss at that moment what was really going on. Why that might have been was anybody's guess. Even I would have been hard-pressed to explain my feelings. So how could my parents know?

This is how the investigation behind Understanding often goes. We're not catching someone at their best moment. It may be a time of terrible suffering and shame. It would be hard to expect lucid, coolheaded analysis from anyone, especially from a child who doesn't yet have a developed emotion vocabulary or the ability to articulate complex feelings while still experiencing them. Every parent has been through this and knows exactly what I'm talking about.

The situation gets worse when adults misinterpret emotional information—say, humiliation rather than malice—and act only on the most conspicuous evidence. Recognizing that something is wrong is only the first step. The skill of Recognition is most valuable for the information it supplies to help us begin to understand what is really happening underneath.

An emotional outburst signals that something is going on, but it doesn't tell us *what*. We need to grant the permission to feel, and then ask the right questions, if we wish to know what's behind that outburst.

Put yourself in the place of a second-grade teacher. Two of your students, Ian and Leila, are working together on a science project. It sits, nearly finished, on Leila's desk.

All of a sudden, Ian jumps up from his seat, takes a swing at Leila's desk, shouts in her face, "I hate you!" and stomps out of the classroom. Their project flies across the room.

Leila picks up the ruined project and starts crying.

You're not going to have an easy time calming either child down and asking the questions necessary to figure out what just happened and why. So all you can do is guess. How must poor Leila be feeling? Ian was belligerent, even violent—what brought that on? It seems clear who was the aggressor and who was the victim.

If you were their teacher, the first thing you might do is help Ian calm down and then ask him to apologize. Nothing Leila did could excuse his outburst. And you'd be right—if your main goal was to teach them both a lesson in social skills and what is acceptable versus unacceptable classroom behavior. This is the kind of sudden explosion that happens in classrooms all the time, just as it happens in homes, among siblings. Our first impulse is to restore order so we can go on with our lives.

This is a critical moment in our attempts to understand emotions. It's easy to get this part wrong. We focus on behavior rather than on what might have caused it. It's like treating the symptom and not the disease. As a result, the best we manage to do is modify behavior—by force. And this distracts us from the underlying causes.

Had we been able to restrain our impulse to control and punish, what might we have done differently in that classroom? Certainly behavior such as Ian's has to be addressed. But rather than cast one child as the wrongdoer and the other as the innocent victim, we might have withheld judgment and talked to them separately, asking a few simple questions: What happened? How are you feeling? And: Why do you feel that way?

Had their teacher done that, and then pursued the answers through as many follow-up questions as it took, she might have learned something interesting.

Ten minutes before Ian's explosion, the children were playing at recess. In front of all the other kids, Leila announced that Ian wets the bed. Even worse, she revealed that the source of her information was the boy's little sister.

To some, that still might not make a difference—Ian was in the wrong no matter how humiliated he felt. But punishing him or making him apologize did nothing about what caused the incident. If we had gotten to the root of Ian's anger, we might have helped him find another way to respond to similar provocations in the future. And if there was a reason Leila did what she did, we'd try to deal with that too.

Understanding requires the use of our storytelling ability, perspective-taking skills, and pattern seeking to piece together the concatenation of feelings and events that led to the current situation. It begins with being an emotion scientist, not a judge. If you aren't asking questions, you haven't acquired the skill yet. If you aren't listening to the answers, you aren't *using* the skill. The emotion scientist has a genuine desire to understand and acknowledges that all emotions are information. Until we understand the *causes* of emotion, we'll never really be able to help ourselves, our kids, or our colleagues.

Had either my mother or father been able to cope with my tantrums and reach out to me, maybe with a hug or some show of affection and acceptance, who knows how those scenes might have ended? If my mother had said something like "Okay, Marc, I can tell you don't want to talk about Hapkido now, how about if we stop for ice cream on the way home and then watch TV?" perhaps we would have found the space to explore what had happened. Maybe at bedtime, a few gently probing questions might have elicited some honest answers, enough to begin understanding what went wrong and why. But, as I said, it was not to be.

Now, through the lens of the emotion scientist, let's go back to the martial arts test and the aftermath. In the absence of any explanation from that raging child, let's imagine four possible versions of what happened.

In scenario number one, the test itself was legitimate and not to blame. All the blocks, punches, and so on that I was required to perform were understood. But my blocks were not strong enough. The sensei said, "Sorry, Marc, it's clear you put in a lot of effort, but your blocks need work. Another couple of weeks and I think you'll get that yellow belt."

Sounds possible. My emotion: most likely disappointment, and completely understandable.

In scenario two, the sensei comes up to me just before the test and says, "Marc, you've been practicing all this time with your friend Mike, but I can't let you do the test with him." Instead, he says, I'll be taking it with a senior student, one of the toughest in the class.

Also plausible. To me, this would have been completely unfair—he should have told me before so I could have prepared. No surprise that I'm angry. I'm also anxious about what the sensei might decide to do if I come back for the retest.

In scenario three, the sensei throws in a few surprise items, all of which are beyond my skills, and I fail. Could also be true. Again, I'm angry over the injustice of his decision.

In scenario four, I fail the test fair and square, but that's just where the problem begins. In the locker room afterward, while I'm changing back into my clothes, one of my tormentors from school comes up to me and says, "You loser, we knew you'd fail! Wait till tomorrow morning on the bus, we'll see how your yellow belt moves help you then."

Of course, how could my mother know which, if any, of those had been the case? She couldn't, unless she began the arduous process of asking the right questions, listening to the answers without judging them, without challenging them, and instead letting them sink in. And then asking more questions.

My tantrum made that unlikely.

Do you see the value of being an emotion scientist in a situation like this? Each emotion has what psychologist Richard Lazarus termed a "core relational theme"—a meaning. The only way to get at the meaning of an emotion is to learn the *why*—how someone perceived the situational factors that produced it. Behavior alone is a clue to the riddle, not an answer.

Let's look again at the four scenarios of my martial arts disaster and search for the underlying themes.

In scenario one, the core meaning of the experience was "unmet expectations." The result was disappointment.

Scenario two's core meaning was "uncertainty"—hence, anxiety.

Scenario three's core meaning was "unfairness"—thus, anger.

Scenario four's core meaning was "impending danger"—hence, fear—and "diminished self-worth"—hence, shame.

Knowing the core relational themes provides critical information about how to understand the emotion. It also helps us figure out how to label, express, and manage what we feel. Think about it: Would the strategies you would use to support your child vary depending on the emotion she or he was feeling? Most likely yes.

Had you known your child was disappointed, you might have helped practice the moves that needed work for the next time.

Had you detected the anxiety, you could have suggested strategies to calm your child's nerves, like a breathing or visualization exercise.

If your child was angry because of unfair treatment, you could have approached the teacher to see if anything could be done differently.

If your child was afraid of being physically beaten the next day, an immediate action was needed—a talk with the principal or bus monitor.

If your child had felt shame, it's possible that professional counseling was needed.

My truth that day was a scenario four. Does knowing this change anything? You might say no. It was unacceptable for me to behave as

I did. I won't disagree. But I can't regulate my reactions until I know what I feel. And it will be hard to do that if the adults who are raising me don't model the skills first or ask the right questions.

Can you imagine how much miscommunication is caused by the inability to see behavior as simply a signal for emotions? This is why we have to be emotion scientists and not emotion judges.

As I started by saying, Understanding is in some ways the most challenging skill to acquire. It calls on all our powers of analysis to honestly and correctly answer that powerful three-letter question: *Why?* Once we ask it, of our own reasons for feeling something or of someone else's, we begin a line of inquiry that can go on for some time. What caused this emotion? Once we find an answer, the next question instantly arises: Why, of all the possible reactions, *that* particular one? At some point we need to feel as though we've answered that original *Why?* But if we stop short, we may never understand our emotions. Sometimes, granted, it takes real bravery to follow the investigation to the end. That's when our skills make us scientists. And paired with genuine motivation, this skill empowers us to be better friends, family members, students, colleagues, and partners.

Now that we've learned how to understand an emotion, we're ready to move on to the next step: labeling it.

6

L: Labeling Emotion

"How are you feeling today?"

That's how I began a talk I recently gave before a group of businesspeople in Napa Valley. At a winery, of course.

Like most of my audiences, nearly all the participants had trouble finding more than a word or two to describe their emotions. As usual, "fine" and "good" were the most popular answers. I tried to dig deeper. There was no deeper. A few broke all the way through to "curious" and "intrigued."

Instead of pressing for reasons why they had such difficulty describing their feelings, I took this group in a different direction.

"Given your expertise," I said, "I'm curious: How do you describe the red wines you're representing?"

Suddenly, these emotional illiterates sounded like poets.

"Rich spice and mineral accents."

"Smoky roasted meat and floral blackberry aromas."

"Bold, supple flavors of apricot and licorice."

"Pepper and cigar box notes."

"Tannins that are big but polished."

"Well-structured, sinewy finish."

"Balanced and driven, with a long finish that lets the fruit echo."

"Dense tannins with a mouth-coating impression."

"Approachable, but built for the cellar."

Can you imagine being so eloquent about fermented grape juice but so limited in describing your inner life?

In recent years there's been discussion of a "vocabulary gap" between rich and poor families. Children growing up in higher-income environments are exposed to more words than their poorer counterparts, and this gap may help account for future educational performance, earning power, even intelligence.

That gap fades when it comes to the words we use to describe our feelings. There, ignorance is egalitarian. There are hundreds of words we could use to describe our feelings, but most of us use one or two: "fine" or "busy."

The question at the core of this book—"How are you feeling?"—doesn't get very far if we don't have any useful answers. Without a proper vocabulary, we can't label our emotions, and if we can't label them, we can't properly consider them or put them into perspective. This isn't just rhetoric. We know from neuroscience and brain-imaging research that there is real, tangible truth to the proposition that "if you can name it, you can tame it." Labeling an emotion is itself a form of regulation. We'll dive more deeply into this science later.

The Recognition chapter was about determining our overall emotional state and locating it on one of the four colored quadrants—red, blue, yellow, or green. The chapter on Understanding was devoted to a single word: *Why?* We talked about the skill of discovering what causes our feelings. Labeling is where we take those two skills to the next level. Here's where we zero in on exactly the emotions we're experiencing, to the point where we can name them precisely.

Are you in the red? Sorry to hear, but now we can determine exactly *where* in the red you are. Are you enraged or merely frustrated?

Frightened or simply concerned? Or, if you're in the green, are you secure or complacent? Blissful or content?

Quite a difference in those emotions, each with its own cause and requiring its own course of action. This is why the Mood Meter is such an important tool: we start with a quadrant, visualized as a basic color, and then narrow the search for a particular shade. This isn't just a device to help us visualize emotions—it's how we discover and label which emotions we're truly experiencing.

In the arc formed by the RULER process, L—Labeling—is the pivot point, the hinge. It connects Recognition and Understanding with Expression and Regulation, which is where we take the actions necessary to draw strength from our emotion lives. Without Labeling, our feelings remain inchoate. Once we name them, we begin to possess their power.

The Labeling skill exists in that space between our understanding of what we feel and our ability to describe it accurately to ourselves and others. When we use the same few emotion words over and over, we revert to that near-mute teenage state of being. Do we really *not* want to know our true feelings? Do we really *not* want other people to understand how we feel? Is this how our fear of vulnerability manifests itself? If you ask me how I feel and I say, "Fine," it spares me having to tell my tale of weakness and woe. "Fine" becomes our polite way of saying, "Please don't ask me how I feel." If I say "Fine" often enough, and you say it often enough, anything more descriptive will seem unnatural—even alarming. But our feelings shouldn't alarm us.

Often, instead of accurately naming our emotions, we'll use figures of speech. I'm on top of the world. You're burned up. He's happy as a clam. I'm down in the dumps. She's blue. All highly evocative, of course. But still, they allow us to evade having to confront, plainly and exactly, what we feel. These inventive metaphors may be descriptive on the written page, but they often create distance between our feelings and our words.

Labeling our emotions with precise words does four main things:

- It legitimizes and organizes our experiences. When we attach a word to a feeling, it gives emotion substance and creates a mental model of the word, which means it can be compared with other feelings we have and also with other people's feelings.
- It helps others to meet our needs. Once we are able to communicate, with specificity, what we're feeling, the people in our lives can look beyond our behaviors to understand their causes. Now, empathy is more available.
- Similarly, it helps us to meet the needs of others. Once we know how someone is feeling, it's easier for us to support them.
- Finally, it connects us to the rest of the world. Our emotions become a form of communication, a way to share the experience of being alive. There's a body of research showing the health benefits of social connectivity, and this is where it begins—in being able to identify with one another. The terminology of emotion allows us to read one another's lives, almost as we would in a novel. The words give us each a story to tell.

That's the power of Labeling.

There are, it is said, around two thousand words in the English language that broadly refer to emotion. That's a lot of possibilities, which makes sense considering the variety of emotions and feelings we all experience in the course of a day.

But then there's the question of how many of those words we actually use. And that's where our attitudes toward emotion begin to peek through our language. To put it bluntly, our emotion vocabulary is woefully insufficient.

For the most part, the emotions that require the most attention, the ones that tend to preoccupy us, are the negative ones—the variations on anger, fear, sadness, and shame. Studies show that feeling words are about 50 percent negative, 30 percent positive, and 20 percent neutral. But even this doesn't mean we're good at describing our negative emotions. We don't like to dwell on unpleasant feelings. We just want them to go away—preferably on their own, without any engagement on our part. Whether they're our own negative emotions or someone else's, they're painful to deal with.

One possible explanation for the preponderance of words defining negative emotions is that our brains process positive and negative feelings differently. We tend to give our positive emotions superficial attention only; we see no need to modulate them, just cross our fingers and hope they last. We don't expend much mental energy analyzing why we feel so good.

But we experience negative emotions more deeply—they slow our processing down because they indicate a problem. Out of necessity we devote more words to their description. Back when my uncle Marvin was building what he called his "Feeling Words Curriculum," he would talk about things such as alienation, deprivation, and other dark feelings, and educators freaked out—they were scared by the idea that children might actually experience such things. But kids *do* have negative feelings frequently, he insisted, and we can either discuss them or ignore them. He didn't get very far with that argument in the 1970s and 1980s, but he was right then and right now.

It's instructive to witness how our understanding of emotion progresses as our brains develop, starting right after birth. Researchers have found that infants are unable to perceive distinct emotions by facial expressions—but they *can* differentiate between pleasant, unpleasant, and neutral expressions. Two-year-olds who know only the most basic emotion words *sad* and *happy* can't tell the difference between negative facial expressions—they perceive all unpleasant faces as "sad." Three- and four-year-olds begin to grasp the terms *anger* and *fear* and learn to tell one negative expression from another. There's ample research showing that children who can accurately label their feelings enjoy more positive social interactions than kids who cannot, who experience more learning and behavioral problems.

This isn't simply theorizing or conjecture. Matthew Lieberman and his colleagues at UCLA conducted experiments to see if using words to describe feelings (which they refer to as "affective labeling") would moderate distressing emotional experiences—actually ease the pain.

In one study, subjects were shown photos displaying negative emotions. The participants who were asked to label the facial expressions reported less distress than those subjects who simply saw the photos but weren't asked to comment. In another, participants who were identified as having extreme fear of spiders—arachnophobia—were placed in a room with a caged spider. Some subjects used emotion words to describe their feelings in that situation, while others used emotion-neutral words to simply state the facts.

The result? Members of the first group were able to take more steps closer to the cage than the other participants. Additionally, greater use of words such as "anxiety" and "fear" during exposure to the spider was associated with reductions in those emotions. Before the experiments were begun, participants stated that they didn't believe Labeling would be an effective emotion regulation strategy. But they were wrong. Lieberman referred to this as "incidental emotion regulation," because the subjects were not aware that Labeling had reduced the unpleasantness.

Other research has shown that affective labeling is linked to lower activation of the amygdala, the brain region that's activated when we feel negative emotions, and higher activation in the right ventrolateral prefrontal cortex (RVLPFC), which supports emotion regulation. And just as our brains make use of neural pathways to connect one region to another, our emotions travel on pathways too. If we're disposed to anger, then certain kinds of stimuli will routinely trigger it, and anger becomes our immediate, go-to response. But if we are able to define multiple shades of that low-pleasantness, high-energy emotion—such as annoyed, disgusted, irritated, frustrated, and so on—then we can modulate our responses and in doing so stop ourselves before we hit full-blown rage at every provocation. Every possible term becomes a moment to pause for self-reflection: Am I feeling it *this* strongly or perhaps something not quite so extreme?

The term *granularity* provides a useful way of thinking about how we label our emotions. All it means is that we define what we feel as precisely and narrowly as words allow—down to the grains—rather than settle for the generalized terms we tend to lean on. Psychologist Lisa Feldman Barrett wrote, in *The New York Times*, that what she calls *emotional granularity* is the "adaptive value of putting feelings into words with a high degree of complexity"—complexity that mirrors our inner lives. In her experiments, participants who were deemed *granular* were better able to differentiate their emotional experiences. Subjects who were low in granularity—called *clumpers*—were less skilled at differentiating emotions (e.g., angry, worried, frustrated). When the two groups were compared, she reported, granular individuals were less likely to freak out or abuse alcohol when under stress and more likely to find positive meaning in negative experiences. They also were better at emotion regulation—moderating their responses in order to achieve desired outcomes. The clumpers, on the other hand, scored worse on those counts, tending to be physically and psychologically ill at a higher rate than the granular crowd.

There's even a term for people who have the slimmest vocabulary to describe emotions: *alexithymia* (the term also refers to the difficulty in recognizing and expressing emotions). One study examining the brains of alexithymic people found that they had less gray matter than non-alexithymic people in areas of their anterior cingulate cortex that are associated with language processing.

It's hard to overstate the connection between the emotions we feel and the words we use to describe them. The Sapir-Whorf hypothesis, named for a pair of linguists, maintains that the language we speak determines our worldview and even how our minds work. This hearkens back to a nineteenth-century idea that language expresses the spirit of a culture. Those beliefs have fallen somewhat out of favor, but scholars are still studying the ways in which language influences thought and the way we experience the world.

The Inuit of Alaska and Canada have dozens of words for snow, or so the popular belief holds. The rest of us make do with just a few. The implication seems clear: the importance of a subject is demonstrated by the number of words available to describe it.

There are emotion words in other languages that don't exist in English. Does this mean that the feelings themselves don't arise among the English-speaking population? Possibly not—it seems unlikely that we're unable to experience certain emotions just because we don't have a single word for them. But the fact that those terms don't appear in our vocabulary must be indicative of something. Anna Wierzbicka, a Polish linguist, contends that we rely too heavily on the English language, which might actually keep us from attaining greater self-awareness.

One word that gets a lot of attention in psychology textbooks describes the feeling of happiness or satisfaction caused by someone else's misfortune, or what is known in German as *schadenfreude*. There are supposedly words with similar meaning in Dutch, Arabic, Hebrew, Czech and Finnish, but no such term in English. Does this mean we're less likely to enjoy seeing someone suffer or that those other nationalities are more malicious than we Anglophones? Maybe it just means they are more comfortable owning up to such a nasty sensation.

That's not the only emotion word that appears in other languages but not in English. Here are a few more:

Litost is a Czech word meaning, according to the novelist Milan Kundera, "a state of torment created by the sudden sight of one's own misery."

Iktsuarpok is the Inuit word that describes the anticipation you feel when you're so impatient for a guest's arrival at your home that you keep going outside to check.

Hygge is the fabled Danish sensation experienced while sitting around a fire in winter surrounded by friends.

Kvell is the Yiddish word that describes the feeling of overwhelming love and pride you get when you see what your child can do.

And *ya'arburnee* is Arabic for "May you bury me"—meaning, the hope that you will die before a loved one because you couldn't stand to live without him or her.

Is there any significance to these differences? In all likelihood, the existence of these terms is in some way a reflection of their cultural patrimony. The words we use are dependent on our values.

On the other hand, there's no word for *emotion* in Tibetan, Tahitian, Bimin-Kuskusmin, Chewong, or Samoan. Presumably, people who speak those languages still have feelings.

But is there really a connection between what we're capable of feeling and what we're able to express? You might think not—even if we never named one of our feelings, we all experience the same set of emotions, don't we? Can our ability to feel be influenced by our vocabulary?

To some degree, it can. If we can acknowledge only the basics that every child knows—*I'm mad, I'm happy, I'm scared, I'm sad*—we're missing a lot of information.

The number of English words and associations for "shame" is no match when compared with the Chinese. In Mandarin, there were more than one hundred different shame-related terms and phrases found in one research article.

In that same spirit, we have to assume that there's a connection between the size of our emotion vocabulary and the importance of emotions in our lives. The more words we can use to describe what we feel, the better able we'll be to understand ourselves and to make ourselves understood to others. And if our counterparts, too, have robust emotion vocabularies, it will be much easier for us to understand them— not just to empathize but also to help them, when needed, to regulate and modulate the feelings they experience.

This, as you can imagine, is of huge importance when dealing with children. Their emotional lives are often a mystery to us precisely because they haven't yet learned to process and express what they feel.

The more words that children can use, the better able we'll be to support them. When we use a wide variety of terms to describe emotions, our children learn the words, but they also absorb the lesson that describing their feelings is a natural, positive thing to do.

Attaching the correct label to the emotion is critical because once we've labeled a feeling, we've also begun figuring out what to do about it. If we assume incorrectly that our child is feeling anxious, we'll fail to address the actual emotion—perhaps embarrassment, maybe fear, both of which can look a lot like anxiety from the outside. Imprecise Labeling can lead us astray as we search for ways to resolve negative emotions.

And that's why emotion vocabulary—Labeling—matters so much.

So it's plain to see the advantages of acquiring (and using) a robust emotion vocabulary. But we haven't yet discussed how we acquire this skill.

One way is simply by using the Mood Meter, which is like a map of emotions. If we refer to it often enough, we may begin to adopt some of the terms as our own. The Mood Meter attempts to cover all the bases of each emotion category: In the upper left red quadrant, it goes from *peeved* to *enraged*, from *uneasy* to *panicked*. The green reaches from *at ease* to *serene*, from *calm* to *balanced*. The blue goes from *down* to *despair* and *lonely* to *alienated*. And the yellow moves from *joyful* to *ecstatic* and *hopeful* to *optimistic*. The full Mood Meter with one hundred words appears on the endpapers. In collaboration with HopeLab, we've also developed an app (www.moodmeterapp.com) so you can track your emotions over time.

In RULER, we teach children emotion concepts using our Feeling Words Curriculum with a goal that by middle school every child will learn a minimum of eighty-four terms that describe, specifically, things they feel. It teaches them the words, and by doing so it also emphasizes the value of acknowledging and accepting the full range of emotions. That lesson is as important as the vocabulary itself.

When we use a general, undefined term to describe how we feel—
"lousy," "fine," "mad"—we make it challenging for anyone to help us.
It could require a lot of investigation to figure out that "lousy" actually
means "I'm *disappointed* because my presentation was not well received
and I thought I aced it" or "I'm *afraid* to tell my colleagues that my
presentation was not well received because they'll blame me for not
being prepared." The more skilled we become at labeling what we feel
and describing why, the more likely we are to get the empathy or help
we need. The ability to accurately label our feelings cuts the rest of the
world a break.

The trick in Labeling is to make sure we've hit on the correct word.
If we go too far afield here, we may find ourselves addressing a problem
that doesn't exist and ignoring one that does. When we become emotion scientists, we find quite a few of these potential near misses that
can lead us astray if we're not attentive.

A challenge with labeling emotions that's common today, in both
our classrooms and our workplaces, is the one centered on what everyone simply calls "stress." When we probe with our questions, we usually uncover at least four possible—separate—emotions: anxiety, fear,
pressure, and stress. At first they seem almost interchangeable, but in
fact they are distinct feelings, each with its own source.

Anxiety, as we learned earlier, is worry about future uncertainty and
our inability to control what will happen to us.

Fear is the palpable sense of a danger that lies just ahead and will
eventually strike at us.

Pressure is the force from the outside that tells us something important is at stake, and whether we succeed or fail will depend on how we
perform.

And, finally, stress is what we feel when we're facing too many demands from all of the above and fear we may not be up to it.

All interconnected feelings, certainly, but distinctly different. Each
has its own underlying theme and cause, and we must first untangle
them if we're to understand them and eventually figure out what to do

about them. Some of the causes are internal, others are intrusions from the outside world.

It's also entirely possible that stress is masking a completely different emotion. I asked a couple hundred students at Yale about their "stress" and learned that it was mostly related to envy. Envy? They would see fellow students getting an A without studying, securing great job offers because of their parents' connections, and so on. I wonder how many college counseling offices are helping kids manage their envy as opposed to offering "stress reduction"?

About ten years ago I suffered with acid reflux and anxiety and blamed it on my neuroses. I lived in a constant low-level dread of the immediate future, and when I went to my doctor he said, "Welcome to Yale." Then he said, "Take some Prilosec and I'll prescribe you some Ativan to alleviate the stress." I wasn't expecting that and left determined to figure out the problem on my own. Was I really stressed or anxious, or was I feeling something else instead?

Finally, I realized that I felt "stressed" because I was taking on too many tasks—more than anyone could easily complete. Stress wasn't the root of my problem—I was overwhelmed. I had too much on my plate. When I cut back a little on my work obligations, scheduled exercise and downtime, my stress levels subsided considerably. I couldn't have come up with that fix if I hadn't been able to analyze exactly what I was feeling, and that began with naming it.

In chapter 5 we discussed jealousy and envy, which are often confused. They're not interchangeable terms, and if we treat them the same, we're going off course. Recall, jealousy is a relationship-driven emotion. It has to do with feeling threatened that you will lose the attention of someone important to you. This could be any relationship—one kid feels like Mom or Dad is spending more time with a sibling, or two work colleagues are at odds because the boss favors one over the other, or it could also be the typical romantic triangle. Envy, on the other hand, has to do with coveting something that someone else possesses. Could be an object but could also be a relationship, an attitude, someone's skill or talent, a frame of mind. If we can't tell any two emotions apart, how are we going to address them and resolve them?

Often, I'll ask audiences to define the difference between anger and disappointment. I'm always surprised to see that people have such a hard time with that one. Most of them say they can't really put the difference into words, which speaks volumes about our difficulty with the vocabulary of emotion. But, as we've said before, anger is usually a response to unfair treatment or an injustice. Disappointment is about an unmet expectation. The strategies we might use to deal with our own or another's disappointment likely would be different from those we'd use for ire.

One of our RULER trainers was having dinner at home with his family when one of his sons began acting out. The boy's mother asked him, "Why are you so angry?" The boy's older brother, who was in a classroom where RULER is implemented, said, "Mom, I don't think Jeremy is angry, I think he's disappointed. He was hoping to go outside to play, but now that it's raining, he can't." Both parents' jaws dropped. They were both extremely conversant in the RULER system but were startled—pleasantly so—to see it in action at their dinner table.

Another common mistake is waiting so long to identify our feelings that they become daunting. We skip over *irritated* or *nervous* or *apprehensive* and, left unattended, they turn into *livid* or *panicked*. We ignore *apathetic* or *drained* until they metastasize into *hopeless* or *depressed* and we're forced to deal with them. We also tend to talk exclusively about our negative emotions, but why not explore our feelings of serenity or cheerfulness? If we never acknowledge those emotions, we may go through life with the sense that we never really experience them. Also, if we devote time and thought to our positive moments, we may discover ways to extend them.

Giving kids awareness of what *peeved* or *irritated* feels like and what thoughts they are having around those feelings is a strategy in itself for preventing outbursts and outbreaks of violence at the extreme ends. If they can recognize a difficult internal state while it's still manageable, kids can get support before they are overwhelmed and unable to regulate. Labeling short-circuits the kinds of spirals that end in tears or tantrums.

A teacher we were coaching in New York City who worked in a school for children with emotional challenges demonstrated this problem. When we first interviewed her, she reported that her students' emotions came out mainly in the extreme—like the enraged kids who threw a desk, or beat up a fellow student, or broke down hysterically crying in class; or the children who were silent but despondent and seriously depressed. Her strategies for dealing with all these situations was to call in the intervention team. But she felt unable to do anything before matters reached the breaking point. As a result, she was routinely the object of their outbursts, even their violence. She went years without reporting the welts and bruises she suffered from blows she received almost daily— because she didn't want her kids to be expelled or go to prison.

Then we introduced the Mood Meter to her school. For the first time, it gave those children a way to become aware of what they were feeling before they erupted into violence and other extreme behaviors. Once they had *irritated* and *frustrated* and *annoyed* in their vocabulary, they were able to acknowledge what was going on before it zoomed all the way to *enraged*. They could explain to their teacher what they were feeling and ask for help while that was still a possibility.

"After a year of using the Mood Meter," she told us, "I had no more welts. The need for intervention decreased. Kids could tell the difference between a little bit of anger and a lot. When they felt a little bit of anger, they could raise their hand and I or the assistant teacher would support them with a strategy to shift before it got out of control. With practice, many students internalized the strategies and used them independently both in class and outside of school."

Bit by bit, the kids took control of their own emotional destinies, without ignoring or silencing what was going on inside. Research shows that a large percentage of children with language impairment exhibit emotional and behavioral problems. But, as we've discussed, when you can name and understand a specific emotion, your brain circuits and nervous system will calm you down. Language skills facilitate executive control and metacognitive processing. Thus, the simple act of acknowledgment creates a shift, and change becomes possible.

I have witnessed the immense power of Labeling firsthand in my own family, not with a child per se but with my dad. When he was seventy-eight, I got an email from his wife, Jane:

"Hi Marc, I wanted to make you aware that I am having problems with Dad. His rages seem more frequent and so is his verbal abuse. I am at the end of my rope. I think he needs medication or maybe a therapist. He, of course, thinks his rages are justified and I am sure he will be extremely mad if he knows I told you. Right now, he gets really mad when I babysit my grandson. I don't do it often, but I love to watch him. I am thankful that I am healthy enough to take care of him once in a while. I don't know what your father's problem is, but I never know when he will explode. I am worn down living this way. I thought maybe you could help. Thank you."

I immediately called my brothers. Of course, our initial conversation brought us all back to our stormy childhood.

We decided to take a road trip to chat with our dad. We had to do this carefully because Jane was afraid of how our dad would respond. We didn't want our visit to backfire on her. We took him out for coffee and brought up Jane's email. Like good emotion scientists, we investigated and looked for cues. I said, "Dad, what's going on with you and Jane? She's really upset about how you are treating her."

"I can't take it anymore," he said.

"What can't you take anymore?" I asked, and then trotted out all the emotion scientist questions, carefully crafting them so as not to offend.

"What's going on?"

"Tell me more."

"What's making you angry?"

"What is Jane doing?"

"When do you get these feelings?"

Here's what he said:

"Her daughter is using her, dropping off her grandson for hours on end. She's spending *so* much time taking care of her grandson. I didn't expect my retirement was going to be spent like this."

I had a hunch, based on the emotion themes coming out of my father's mouth, that he wasn't so much angry as he was jealous of the grandson who was getting all his wife's attention.

To be sure, he resented her children, too, for how much they were relying on her. But the core theme was that he felt threatened by the grandson because Jane seemed to prefer to be with him, leaving my dad alone.

So I said, "Dad, it seems like you might be jealous of Jane's grandson."

He looked at me as if I were nuts.

Then I said, "Well, it seems like you want to spend more time with Jane, and you're not happy with the fact that she's spending so much time with her grandson. That's jealousy."

"Are you telling me I'm jealous?" he said.

"No," I said, "*you're* telling me you're jealous."

At that point, my dad started crying. He suddenly realized what he was actually feeling. He felt threatened by a little kid.

Now we had an opening to make a change. We had created a space to help my father manage his feelings.

That day transformed the lives of my dad and his wife. About a month later, Jane called and said, "Marc, I have no idea what you did that day, but whatever it was, it worked. Thank you. He's *different*!"

When you can understand and name your emotions, something magical happens. The mere fact of acknowledgment creates the ability to shift. When we don't have the words for our feelings, we're not just lacking descriptive flourish. We're lacking *authorship* of our own lives.

After the challenges of U—Understanding emotions—Labeling should feel like a break. We all know plenty of words that describe emotions, feelings, and moods. Even if we don't normally use them in connection with our own lives, we read them and hear them all around us. A great deal of life is defined by words such as *ecstatic, anxious, furious, content, dubious, hopeful, acquiescent*. Any thesaurus or dictionary can handle that part of this skill. Our job then becomes just to begin affixing those commonplace terms to what we're feeling inside. When we settle for the six or seven words that we all rely on, we're short-changing ourselves—it's like taking a vow of emotional poverty when riches await. Ask yourself now: How am I feeling? And try coming up with as many words—more thoughtful and precise ones than you usually deploy. That's how this skill improves. Without it, we remain unknown to ourselves or anyone else, which brings us to our next step: expressing emotion.

7

E: Expressing Emotion

RATHER THAN ASK HOW you're feeling (again!), I'll just say I hope you're feeling brave.

The three previous chapters required us to learn valuable emotion skills. Recognizing our own feelings and those of other people. Understanding the causes and consequences. Labeling those emotions precisely.

Those steps have something important in common: they're about the inner experience of emotions. Digging deep into feelings isn't always easy, but there's not much external risk involved.

With this chapter, that changes. With Expression, we reveal ourselves. Now we'll have to decide: *Can I share this?*

And if the answer is yes, then how much exactly do we share, and when, and where, and with whom? Do I let my mom/dad, colleague, friend, significant other, child, know what I'm really feeling and why? It can be terrifying—as it was for me to share what was happening in my childhood. The abuse, the bullying. Before we express our emotions, we can't help but wonder: Will I be heard? Accepted? Judged? Will I get the support I need? Will I get disowned? Am *I* even ready to own these feelings?

E can be the scariest of the five letters, because here's where we take what we've discovered in RUL—the intimate things we've learned about ourselves—and begin to do something about them.

This could be a sensitive moment, depending on what we have to express and to whom we're about to express it. On the one hand, it's important to be honest and forthcoming. On the other, we need to take the possible consequences of our honesty into account. In a sense, expressing emotions is like a transaction between people. You express, and I react. In that back-and-forth, we may come to understand each other and be better off for it. But the opposite could also be true—your emotions might provoke something negative in me, something I'm not prepared to deal with or control. In which case, honest expression has the potential to distance us or make both our lives significantly worse, at least in the short run. We need the sensitivity to balance one thing with another.

Looking back, I realize that the inability to express emotion was at the center of all my childhood trauma. Had I been able to tell my parents the horrible things I was feeling—fear, anxiety, shame—then they would have discovered the source of all those destructive emotions. They would have heard about the sexual abuse I endured in secret and the bullies who victimized me every day at school. It isn't only feelings that we hide—it's what is causing them.

Today, this comes up often regarding the women, men, and children who have been sexually abused or harassed and yet never uttered a word or called out their abusers. It's no secret why—many believed their feelings of shame and guilt would be even more unbearable once they were out in the open. Others might not share because they don't think anyone would believe them or because of fear of retaliation. The inability to express those emotions is like a continuous pain that lingers on. In a way, the silence is as damaging as the assault itself.

In my childhood, the causes of my emotional pain were overwhelming to me, but they were mostly things my parents or teachers could have helped me to manage. I might have been spared a world of torment—if only I had felt free to say what I was feeling.

Instead, I tortured myself with questions: How will they react if I tell them? What will they think of me? Will they be angry or disappointed in me? What will they do in response—blame me, ignore me, shame me? For whatever reasons, I didn't have permission to feel at home or at school, so my emotions remained bottled up inside, leading to self-doubt, low self-worth, extreme loneliness.

And when my feelings did boil over—as they always do—they often came out as fury I was unable to articulate. My behavior only made things worse. I knew of no other way to express myself.

In elementary school, those pent-up feelings turned into physical pain—I began suffering with a mysterious gastrointestinal ailment that defied all attempts to diagnose it. That's because there likely *was* no physiological cause of my illness. It was the result of emotional suffering that had no other way out. The pain *was* my form of expression. And in middle school my unexpressed emotions turned into self-hatred and an eating disorder.

I've been describing the negative emotions that plagued me as a child. And it's true that feelings such as shame, jealousy, anxiety, and so on are the hardest ones to express. But we also have trouble making our positive feelings known to others. Perhaps we don't want to sound as though we're bragging or gloating. Maybe it's because happiness doesn't require empathy from other people—it's its own reward in that sense. But it's equally important to know how to label all our positive emotions and make them known to the people who are closest to us. It's part of what keeps us close.

During those times when we suffer in silence, we make it impossible for anyone to truly know us, understand us, empathize with us, or—the big one—help us. When we suppress those feelings, we send a message to everyone in our path: I'm fine even when I'm not. Stay back. Keep your distance. Don't ask why, because I don't want to tell you what's going on.

But when we express our emotions, we're saying:

Here's what I feel and why.

Here's what I want to happen next.

Here's what I need from you right now.

It's probably as intimate as we'll ever be.

In public settings, I'll frequently ask educators, "How many of you are in the yellow or green quadrant?" Nearly everyone will raise a hand. Then I tell them that in our confidential surveys, people report being in the red or blue quadrant roughly 60 to 70 percent of the time. Mostly positive feelings when I ask in public, mainly negative when we pose the question privately.

You can't really fault people for this. We all do it. It's human nature. Who wants to look like the emotional oddball—the sad, anxious, depressed, angry one in a crowd of people claiming to be upbeat and optimistic? We have a natural bias in favor of displaying positive emotions, especially in the United States, which translates into a pressure on all of us to seem happy no matter what. Which, as it turns out, often backfires and makes us *less* happy.

It's the lie we all tell, meaning it can't be much of a lie, since we're not fooling anybody. But that doesn't stop us.

At a recent talk I gave to more than five hundred business managers and community leaders, after I asked how they were feeling, I said, "Who's willing to share?"

Only two people raised their hands. Instead of trying to coax more, I asked everyone to choose a partner and discuss *why* they thought no one wanted to open up.

"Does anybody *really* want to know how we feel?" asked one.

"Why would we talk about it?" another said. "When you're a woman, talking about your feelings only makes you seem weak."

I go through this same drill with practically every group I meet. I'm forever trying to find reasons we're so reluctant to share how we feel. I'm always learning new ones.

One student told me, "My school is like a prison. Our school rules dictate how we *should* feel, so why would I bother expressing how I really feel?"

A student who was a witness in the Parkland, Florida, shootings said, "I want to share how I feel with my mom, but she's under so much stress I don't want to bother her."

A parent said, "I would never share that I was bullied with my son, he'll think I'm not tough enough to raise him."

Someone I interviewed who works in a tech company said, "In my office, it's not safe to share, people will just gossip."

One high school girl said, "After we lost my brother, my dad shut down and we never talked about my sister's suicide. It just wasn't an option."

A teacher once told me, "I don't share because I'm afraid that once I open up, I'll never be able to close the floodgate."

A high school boy said, "Every time I try to have a conversation, it gets brushed off. My dad says things like 'Don't worry about it. It'll be fine.' What he doesn't know is that I'm *not* fine."

A burned-out teacher recently told me, "If I shared how I felt to all my students, none of them would want to come to class. They'd have no respect for me."

A lawyer in her fifties told me, "I've lived long enough with my husband without sharing, who knows what would happen to our relationship if I start now?"

A lesbian in high school said, "My parents' background makes it really difficult for me to be open. They just don't understand. I can't talk about the girls I want to date. They'll disown me."

Chances are if I were to ask you the same question, your answer would sound a lot like these. We all experience the same emotions, yet we all hide them from one another. It's weird.

Emotional suppression is a major force in schools, and it's not just the students who are discouraged from showing their feelings. An old adage that circulates among teachers tells us, "Don't smile until Christmas," meaning that educators should start out acting like strict, uninviting taskmasters to maintain tight control over their classrooms.

But is that how educators can best demonstrate their standards and expectations? Is smiling—or making any sort of kind, genuine gesture, even telling jokes—going to hinder the educational process? Though it is the responsibility of teachers to maintain sufficient control and set expectations for student performance and behavior, our classrooms are not meant to be *ruled*. Teachers are guides, not dictators. The research is clear: the best way to engage students is to develop relationships, not prevent them, and the currency of relationships is emotional expression.

We've all heard the saying "Children should be seen and not heard." It hearkens back to a time when people actually believed such nonsense. As a society, we've moved beyond that, thankfully. But it's easy to detect the vestiges of that outlook. We tend not to appreciate excessive emotional expression even from children.

"My teacher said I'm not allowed to cry in class," a colleague's six-year-old son told her one day. "She said I have to be a big boy and feel happy at school." This is a result of the idea that happiness is the only acceptable feeling in public, and if we're not happy at all times, we've failed. We're sending our kids this message when they're at their most impressionable. What about the child who is just temperamentally subdued? Or one who is experiencing sadness or struggling at home? That poor kid may have no place else to be emotionally honest.

Because of their still developing vocabularies and powers of communication, we need to listen extra closely to our children if we're interested in knowing what they feel and why. We need to make sure they understand that we welcome hearing what happens in their lives—the good and the bad, the happy and the sad, the successes and the failures.

As infants, before we acquire the language to express emotions, we are helpless to hide them. We're pure emotion, though our feelings may be elemental and our needs limited to a very few practical ones. Researchers have identified the following in the newborn's supply of emotional expressions:

- Interest
- Enjoyment
- Surprise
- Sadness/distress
- Anger
- Discomfort/pain
- Fear
- Disgust

Wordlessly, babies get their messages across loud and clear, as any parent can attest. Infant emotions are focused on the basics of survival—the need for food, sleep, physical comfort, and security. This underscores the primary purpose of emotional expression: it keeps us alive. From a Darwinian perspective, demanding attention to our feelings is a necessity, not a choice.

As we develop and acquire language, our emotional needs become more complex, and so does how we make them known. But paradoxically, as we acquire the power to express our emotions, we also develop the ability (and the desire) to hide them—to obfuscate, to deceive, to deny. It's a trade-off—the more sophisticated we become in our ability to say what we feel, the more control we exert over ourselves. Out of shame? For self-protection? Or do we sense that the people around us wish, for their own reasons, that we should keep at least some of our feelings to ourselves?

As we've said before, it's scary to hear other people express their feelings, because we may have to accept some hard truths about ourselves. And in response, we may feel obliged to take some action—even to change, which is usually the last thing we want to do.

Years ago, I was excited to have my two older brothers come to hear me speak. They're convinced I make a living by sitting around in coffee shops thinking (they are partially right). It was a large presentation to a couple thousand people in a New York hotel auditorium. They sat up front. I kept an eye on them and noticed the look of pleasure and pride on their faces during the first fifteen minutes of the talk. Their facial expressions said: Wow, that's my brother up there!

Then I began telling the audience about the bullying I endured as a child, the anger and anxiety I witnessed in my parents, the "strategies" they used to regulate their own emotions, such as my mother's secret Styrofoam cup filled with Dewar's scotch. I also talked about their more memorable child-rearing tools. Suddenly, my brothers weren't looking so pleased or proud.

After the talk ended, I caught up with them heading toward the exit and asked, "Hey, what did you think?"

"Don't walk out with us," one brother said.

"I can't believe how much you shared about yourself," the other one said. "People are going to think you're *weak*."

I was surprised, but not shocked. They grew up in the same house I did, under the same rules. I knew where they were coming from. I didn't tell them this, but I remember thinking: You guys would both benefit from doing a little more talking about your emotions.

I'm reminded of the old tune "Smile," the lyrics of which convey some real truths about the way we think of emotions, especially the unhappy ones. The song tells us to smile when our hearts are aching and breaking. The clear message is that we should hide our negative feelings—not just hide them but wear a mask to tell the world the exact opposite of the truth. Strangely, there is something utterly heartrending about that sentiment. We are moved by the thought of masking our negative emotions behind a "show of gladness." At some level we find it oddly ennobling when someone hides their unhappiness.

But why?

It's an implicit acknowledgment that, as human beings, our impulse is to sometimes do as the song says and *hide every trace of sadness*—to cover up the emotions we associate with vulnerability and loss and show the world that we're unaffected, at least on the surface.

So how do we square these two sides of ourselves? Is it possible for us to pursue emotional health by expressing the things we feel—*all* the things we feel—without feeling too exposed for comfort?

Picture it: Today is the day you finally worked up the courage to express what you truly feel, fearlessly and with no attempt to hide it, deny it, or couch it in terms meant to comfort others. Maybe for the first time in your adult life, you spoke your heart with utter honesty.

And it felt fantastic—like a cleansing, like a purge. At first, it was scary to vent so completely, with no regard for how it would be received, but you did it. Congratulations.

And as you finished, you looked around to see your spouse packing his or her bags, your kids cowering in the corner, and the dog hiding under the bed—and then your boss calls to say you're fired.

And you wonder, was there a better way of handling this?

We need to clear up a misunderstanding that may have been building in your mind: that permission to feel means license to let it all hang out, to whine, yell, act on every emotional impulse, and behave as though we have no control over what we feel, so we should just go for it and freak out. Some people think of this kind of venting as being authentic. But habitual, unhealthy methods of expression—yelling, gossiping, verbal or physical aggression, among many others—almost always creates havoc in our lives.

Psychologists and social workers use the term *emotional labor* to describe the effort required to manage the way we express our feelings. The sociologist Arlie Hochschild first defined it as creating "a publicly visible facial and bodily display within the workplace" and studied how people in certain professions—nurses, kindergarten teachers, police officers, flight attendants, and any jobs involving customer contact—frequently are required to put on false fronts. Of course, a similar disconnect happens in nonwork settings too—at home, with family and friends, even among the people with whom we are most intimate.

It may not sound like labor in the usual sense, but managing how and when we express emotions does require sustained effort, and it wears us down, especially when there's a big contrast between what we express and what we actually feel. After a while, it begins to feel natural to suppress our true feelings and a little scary to let them show. Research shows that this so-called surface acting leads to burnout, lower job satisfaction, and even increased anxiety and depression.

It should come as no surprise that something as untamed and unpredictable as our emotional selves requires a complex set of regulations governing expression. So we have what are known as "display rules"— the unwritten but widely agreed-upon guidelines for how, where, when, and in whose presence we may express our feelings. As with any unwritten rules, there's quite a bit of nuance and variation, depending in this case on many factors, including culture, gender, race, age, social status, and power—specifically, the power differential.

We all have different expectations and personal rules about how to express our emotions. Many of these rules are fine as long as they don't interfere with our ability to live healthy lives. But a whole lot of these rules are related to stigma, which only holds us back or can even backfire. My father's rule that prevented him from talking to me about his own childhood victimization may have had an internal logic—but it came out in real life as shame and aggression.

Over the years, I've noticed that people have varying levels of comfort expressing their emotions, depending on where they are and whom they're around. Some of us also are unaware when we are actually expressing certain emotions—we think we're masking our true feeling or showing a poker face, but our microexpressions, which can include that subtle fake smile, quick eye roll, or flirtatious gaze into someone's eyes, reveal something very different might be going on underneath.

Expression is generally a co-skill. It's kind of like tennis—you can't really do it alone. If the listener doesn't do her or his part, it's unlikely that anything useful will come of it. How many of us have been on the brink of some seriously emotional moment, and we've looked up to see our loved one checking their email, or posting something on Instagram, or looking out the window, possibly dreaming of escape. This likely is someone who either doesn't care, is addicted to technology, or is fearful that you'll say something they'd rather not hear.

We're all expert at sending the unmistakable signals of indifference. It's in our defensive body language, our lack of eye contact, the subtle vocal inflections, the silences that last just a little too long. At the same time, we all know how much it hurts to have someone refuse to pay attention.

And so a key skill involved in Expression is listening. Not just hearing. We must be conspicuously open, patient, and sympathetic to whatever's being said. No crossed arms. No restless moving around. No looking away. This is also where the difference between the emotion scientist and the emotion judge comes into play. By our responses to what we're hearing—by our words, body language, facial expressions, and eye contact—we send the message *I'm here for you. I'm not judging. I want to understand you and help you.*

Aside from all the personal restrictions we put on ourselves and one another, there are plenty of societal rules for who may and may not express which emotions. These regulations are far from simple and often stem from stereotypes that are themselves damaging. In times of social upheaval, as we are experiencing today, the norms are shifting and evolving. As we've seen, inequality, injustice, and unfairness are generally met with anger—that's how we humans are built. And anger is, in turn, often met with fear. Taken altogether, it makes for a potent mix of discontent and discord, which sounds a lot like the world as it exists today.

In truth, many of the controversies that dominate the news today have their roots in differences in how we experience and express our feelings.

For instance, gender is a major force in determining emotional expression. According to research, women tend to express themselves more overall, particularly positive emotions, and also internalize negative ones such as sadness and anxiety more than men do. Men, on the other hand, tend to express higher levels of aggression and anger than women. But when subjects' physiological signs of emotional excitement, such as blood pressure and cortisol release, are measured, men score higher—indicating that they likely feel as much as women do but keep more pent up inside.

Women make it easier to tell what they're feeling because they're freer with facial expressions, gestures, and vocal tones. Researchers say that while women smile more often than men, that gender divide doesn't begin to appear until children are in middle school. Women have always been expected to smile, which is now part of the ongoing realignment of relations between the sexes—women have begun to reject strangers' exhortations that they smile and instead see these encounters as a form of harassment. Their anger is understandable—the constant pressure to always appear happy is a requirement that doesn't exist for the men who are doing all the urging.

Both genders cry, but women are more apt to do so in the company of family or friends, while men tend to do it alone. Women also report higher empathy than men, which may account, in part, for those tears.

Race is another strong influence.

Minorities report fears that emotional displays will fall into traps set by old stereotypes and trigger a backlash. So African American mothers, in a survey, said that they counsel their sons and daughters to temper their expressions of anger, lest they be judged more harshly than whites. Anger is the usual response to feelings of injustice and unfairness, while fear is the reaction to the imminent possibility of harm. That dynamic can be seen as an unspoken acknowledgment by whites of how unfairly African Americans have been treated. But on the emotional plane, the group most entitled to anger feels least able to express it, while whites enjoy what's known as "anger privilege"—the right to display anger without the worry of being penalized for it.

Another factor in emotion suppression: children who grow up in high-crime neighborhoods are taught to display toughness and unemotionality, regardless of what they're feeling inside. This may serve a short-term purpose—it's a form of self-preservation—but in the long run it can create one more barrier to self-knowledge.

Gender, race, culture, and class together make a potent combination to suppress the expression of certain emotions.

During the 2018 U.S. Open final, Serena Williams was penalized for calling the umpire "a thief" when he took a point from her for smashing her tennis racket. In the past, male players have yelled, screamed, and called umpires names and have not been penalized in a game. That was just the latest example of how male and female anger are perceived differently. This gender gap comes in many forms, and we've heard them all debated in recent years. When men are forceful, they're strong and assertive; when women are, they're called bossy and controlling. When a man raises his voice, everyone snaps to attention; when a woman does, she's dismissed as shrill or hysterical.

Society tells us that when a woman expresses her intense negative emotions publicly, she's lost control and should be penalized. When a man does the same, it's normal male behavior and does not merit punishment. Widely held beliefs, sometimes outside our awareness, align with gender stereotypes and influence how we express our own emotions as well as how we perceive those of others.

If we notice increasingly intense anger expressed by women, African Americans, and other historically disadvantaged groups, we can take that as a positive sign—an indication that we live in a more just society than before. Even if the price of social justice is more anger than ever—at least for some time.

Power inequality is a strong influence.

The workplace is a perfect arena for studying how the power differential decides who may and may not express emotion freely. The chairman of the board and the CEO are invulnerable, so they enjoy relative freedom to display their feelings without fear of overstepping boundaries. They can express certain negative emotions—anger, frustration, irritation—without paying any price. Indeed, making those feelings known may strike fear into subordinates' hearts and bring about desired results.

But employees further down the totem pole might quickly be out of a job for displaying the same emotions. For those workers, expressions of happiness, optimism, and high energy are safer bets. Meanwhile, the boss might be unwise to express sadness, fear, or anxiety, feelings a junior employee can probably get away with. So the sword cuts both ways.

We take it for granted that in a relationship, the person with more power has greater latitude in expressing emotions. Parents get away with displays they'd never tolerate in their children. In the classroom, the teacher is the boss and the children are the bossed, a dynamic that carries over into the workplace, whether we want it to or not. When we are made to deal with police officers, we recognize the wisdom in emotional restraint, no matter what the officer says or (within limits) does. Right at this moment, we have a chief executive who seems to be absolutely unbridled when it comes to emotional expressiveness, while those around him walk on eggshells, doing their best not to provoke his wrath. Many of the worst injustices in contemporary life revolve around the inability of the powerless to express their fear and outrage at inhumane treatment by abusers. So when we discuss whether or not emotions should be expressed, it's not a trivial matter. Sometimes, it's literally life or death.

Culture is another strong influence.

On a global level, display rules become even more of an issue than they are at home. They dictate which emotional expressions are considered appropriate in any given culture, including how we interact. In the United States, where individuality is prized, the custom is to establish eye contact and deal with people in a direct, face-to-face way. When I first traveled to Korea to study martial arts, I was told never to look the master in the eye and to bow in his presence. I may have overdone it—I avoided looking into his face so assiduously that he finally asked me if anything was wrong.

Wallace Friesen conducted some of the original research on the expression of emotion across cultures. In one study, he showed stress-inducing films and neutral films to American and Japanese participants and compared their facial expressions while they watched the films. When the participants in each culture watched the films alone, they both showed virtually the same facial responses. However, when an older, male scientist was present while the participants watched the stress-inducing film, Japanese participants masked negative emotional expressions with smiles more than American participants.

Recent research by Jeanne Tsai, a professor at Stanford University, and her colleagues has revealed that cultures are more likely to express the specific emotions they value. In one study, top-ranked U.S. government officials, executives, and university leaders used more excited-looking smiles than leaders in China. The display of high-arousal positive emotions is often viewed as a violation of social rules in China where there is an emphasis on cohesiveness among individuals and a prioritization of the group over the self. Other research has shown that competitors from more collectivist cultures tend to express more intense shame displays (head drops, postural constrictions) upon losing, which is consistent with the more pronounced emphasis on modesty and not standing out in collectivist cultures.

Consider another way emotional expression varies. Perhaps you have been on a trip and noticed differences in how strangers interact when passing on the street, how friends express affection, or how children show their deference toward adults. Years ago, I traveled to Croatia with my graduate school classmate Zorana, who was born and raised there. One morning I took a walk and noticed that my normal smiles and waves good morning to people on the street were not being reciprocated. After a few unreturned greetings, I even realized that people were pausing to stare at me.

When I returned to the hotel, I asked Zorana what was up. She said that in Croatia people do not generally say "hi" to strangers on the street. But when they do, it means they want to engage you in conversation. So, here I was thinking, Why are people so unfriendly here? while they were thinking, Who is this weirdo who waves and then keeps walking? This was another lesson on how being an emotion judge and not an emotion scientist leads to major misunderstandings.

Cultural differences don't exist just on a global scale. The rules are different in New Haven, Connecticut, than seventy miles away in New York City. On Wall Street, the top guys bond with big grins and bone-crushing handshakes. Here in the genteel Ivy League, many maintain their emotional—and physical—coolness at all times.

Permission to feel can sometimes mean expressing an emotion we *don't* necessarily feel—it's not being dishonest but rather finding a way of communicating that takes other considerations into account.

A few times in my career I've walked out onto a stage to do a presentation in front of thousands of educators while feeling totally despondent. In one case, I had just gotten the news that Uncle Marvin died. I had a few alternatives: I could have canceled my talk; I could have taken the stage and shared my sad news with the group; I could have put on a smile and a stiff upper lip and pretended nothing had happened. These are the kinds of choices we all are forced to consider throughout the day without thinking much about them. For whatever reason, you feel awful. Are you going to unload on everyone you meet? Go into temporary denial and carry on? These strategies are obvious, accessible, and second nature after a while.

In the case of my presentation after Uncle Marvin's death, I had another option: Find a way to perform well, serve the people in the audience who had come to be inspired, and still express and honor the emotions I was feeling. Without mentioning that Marvin had died, I started by dedicating my talk to Uncle Marvin and thought about how elated he would be that our work was reaching ever more people.

I knew that after the talk was over, I would have support from my family and the chance to feel my grief. Which is exactly what happened.

Expression doesn't affect just our emotional lives—there's abundant research into the physical and mental benefits of expressing emotions. And we should keep in mind that expression need not be only of the spoken, face-to-face variety. Sometimes, sharing with other people is too difficult. In those cases, it may be better to express it in writing. Many of us have had the experience of writing something in a journal or letter that seemed impossible to say in conversation.

According to Professor James Pennebaker, of the University of Texas–Austin, keeping secrets can actually make people ill. But when we transform our feelings and thoughts into language, his research has found, our health often improves. ·

Expressing emotions benefits us in these specific ways:

• Significant drops in physician visits
• Increases in immune function
• Lower blood pressure
• Long-term improvement in mood
• Reduction in stress
• Higher grades for college students
• Less absenteeism at work

In one study, Pennebaker divided fifty students into two groups and asked one group to write essays about emotionally significant issues and the other group to write about superficial matters for four consecutive days. When tested months afterward, the first group showed improvements in immune system function and fewer trips to the university's student health center. And even though members of that first group said they felt distress when writing about sensitive subjects, three months later they reported being happier than the other group. Pennebaker concluded that suppressing traumatic experiences is debilitating, while confiding them to someone else, or writing them down, can bring relief.

More good reasons for expressing how we feel.

Now that we've learned something about Expression, I'm wondering: What emotions do you show the most, at home and at work? Are they what you are really feeling or only the ones you feel you're allowed to display? How would your spouse or partner, colleague or boss, or kids rate your expression skills?

Are you comfortable expressing the emotions in each quadrant: yellow, red, blue, and green? What rules have you created about what you'll express to whom? How much emotional labor are you putting in each day? Is it affecting your performance at work, your relationships, your overall well-being?

These are tough questions to answer, I realize. But they're the ones we need to ask ourselves regularly.

What can we do when the fear of stigma chokes off our ability to express? First: Give ourselves and others permission to feel. Accept and acknowledge that there's no shame in expressing our emotions. We don't need to fix or hide what we feel. Expression enhances our lives in many ways, not all of them obvious. It propels us forward, in this case to the final step—Regulation.

8

R: Regulating Emotion

OKAY, SAME OLD QUESTION: How are you feeling? But now I'd also like to know what (if anything) you're going to do about it.

Imagine it's Friday afternoon and you're away from the office at a conference you're required to attend. It's been a long week and you'd give anything to be home, unwinding, or even back at work. Instead, you're stuck in a windowless meeting room, supposedly paying attention, but here's what's going through your head: *I can't believe I have to sit here for three hours and listen to these people talk while I pretend to listen.*

You're irritated. You're distracted. You're tired. Perfectly understandable.

I describe this scenario when I speak before groups and then ask participants to share the strategies they'd use to deal with their feelings. Here's what they say:

"I'll leave my feelings at the door."

"I'm going to sit up front with good posture."

"I'll drink a lot of coffee."

"I'll focus on you and not let anything distract me."

"I'll take good notes."

"I'm just going to stay positive."

"I'm going to get up and stretch or move around once in a while."

"I'll doodle."

"I'm just going to push through it."

"I'll have a cigarette in the parking lot."

Over the last couple of years, these answers have become quite fashionable:

"I'm going to breathe and be present."

"I'm going to be mindful."

"I'll pray for the best."

And here are a few of my personal favorites:

"I can always leave."

"I'm going to stare at the clock."

"It's up to *you* to keep me engaged!"

"I'm giving you five minutes to keep my attention, otherwise I'm going back on Facebook."

"What kind of question is this? I came to hear a talk by a Yale professor. All you're doing is asking us how we manage our feelings. Do your lecture and I'll listen." (You can't make this stuff up!)

But then I ask my audience: Are these strategies really going to help you? Are they so good that you'd teach them to your kids to help them get through similar situations?

Imagine that instead of adults at a work conference, you're one of a bunch of fifth graders filled with all the typical urges and anxieties that children experience. It's Friday afternoon and you're in social studies. Maybe you stayed up late last night working on your science project that was due today, and you're exhausted. Maybe you bombed on a math quiz this morning and you're afraid you're going to flunk and get grounded. Maybe at breakfast today your father told you that he and your mother are getting a divorce, adding, "You'll probably be getting a new stepfather real soon." (That's a real-life one I heard.)

Okay, now let's revisit those adult strategies to see how well they'll work here.

Would you advise children to walk around the classroom at their leisure? To ignore the teacher and go on Instagram? Leave their feelings at the door? Stare at the clock? Challenge the teacher to justify today's lesson?

Are you laughing yet? Will you ever be able to imagine a weary eleven-year-old dragging herself to the coffeepot at the back of the classroom? Or a student who says, "I'm giving myself permission to go back on Snapchat because this lesson is *boring*." And how might the rest of the class respond to a dozen students randomly popping up out of their seats to stretch and walk around the class?

Emotion regulation is at the top of the RULER hierarchy. It's likely the most complex of the five skills and the most challenging. It's nearly impossible to imagine what life would be like without the power to regulate our emotions. You've been doing it since you were born—and you've done it, to some degree or other, every minute of your waking life.

Except that if you're like most of us, you haven't been very good at it. You've been doing it in haphazard, ad hoc, inconsistent ways. Sometimes your attempts to manage your emotions even have done more harm than good. Have you ever just lost your temper and yelled at someone? You almost certainly haven't been doing it consciously, in the most mindful ways, at the appropriate moments, with a positive outcome as your goal.

Every emotional response is a unique experience. What triggers an unpleasant emotion today may not even register tomorrow. Today you're waiting in line at Starbucks for what seems like an eternity, and all you want to do is leap over the counter, grab your coffee out of the barista's hands, and split. Tomorrow, same Starbucks, but your emotional state is serene, so you happily gaze around the place and people-watch while you wait.

This underscores the importance of the first three emotion skills we learned—we need to know what we're feeling and why before we can anticipate which emotion regulation strategies we might require in the next five minutes.

All of which explains why it's so important that we fully understand and master this, our final skill—Regulation.

Up until now, all the RULER skills have been essentially thoughts and words. Now comes the hard part: putting all that wisdom you gathered from the first four RULER skills into action. This is the nuts-and-bolts chapter, where the real work gets done. It's also where the rewards lie.

Stanford University psychology professor James Gross, an authority on emotion regulation, defines it as "the process by which individuals influence which emotions they have, when they have them, and how they experience and express these emotions."

Our center is especially interested in how people develop constructive strategies that promote personal growth, foster and maintain positive relationships, and lead to both greater well-being and goal attainment.

Of all the skills, this is the one with the most moving parts. In a way, that makes it both the easiest and the hardest one to tackle—the number of specific strategies for Regulation is nearly limitless, depending on the situation and the emotions involved. The strategies that work for you today might not work for you tomorrow. And the strategies that work for you might not work for your partner or child.

As I said earlier, our emotions flow in a continuous stream, like a river, and to keep up with that we're constantly regulating them. It's how we maintain our balance and keep from being swept away by one strong feeling or another. We all know people who seem particularly unskilled at regulating their emotions. They're easily knocked off course by their feelings, and routinely overreact in unhelpful ways. Or, at the other extreme, they suppress their emotional responses so much that they seem cold and numb. They don't permit themselves to feel at all, which is just as harmful as reacting in excess.

We start regulating early. Babies suck their thumbs because it provides emotional comfort. Distressed infants will turn their faces away from the source of their displeasure, another rudimentary form of Regulation. So you see, you've been doing it all your life. You just didn't know it was a skill. I never even heard the term *emotion regulation* until I was in graduate school!

The initial goal of Regulation is to manage our own emotional responses, but then this skill makes a leap into even greater complexity: co-regulation. Every human interaction we've ever had, from infancy onward, has involved co-regulation. It's impossible to be in the company of another being and not be influenced by her or his emotional state, and vice versa.

Originally, co-regulation was a term used to describe the back-and-forth between a caregiver and infant to support a baby's stress regulation. Beginning in the earliest days of life, an infant's socioemotional circuitry is molded by adults. A caregiver who reliably provides physical and verbal comfort and reassures the infant teaches it that emotional distress is manageable. A caregiver who does not provide such support teaches the infant that he or she may be at the mercy of their emotions. In this way, co-regulation is the precursor to healthy self-regulation.

In adult relationships, co-regulation can be intentional, as when we speak soothingly to someone who's upset or try to inspire someone into action. You're joyous, or furious, or bored, and I automatically read the signals and my mood is altered. We're all constantly affecting each other's emotional state.

Sometimes we can use this skill to keep colleagues motivated and striving toward a common goal. In 2015, our center collaborated with Born This Way Foundation to host the Emotion Revolution Summit at Yale. The goal was to build awareness of the critical role emotions play in young people's lives. We wanted to bring together youths from around the country for a summit to share their ideas with educators, academics, and policy makers.

Our first order of business was simply to figure out what we wanted to do at the conference. That was the fun part, and Regulation played a big part. During those early brainstorming meetings, we played upbeat, lively music to inspire dynamic, ambitious thinking. As a result, the energy flowed and everybody was psyched and we had a lot of fun coming up with a long list of possibilities. Nothing got shot down, no matter how far out or impractical. The sky was the limit.

Once we had those ideas, it was time to get practical. We needed to begin winnowing the list and agree on how it all would get done and who would be doing what. For these meetings, we again used music to regulate the team's mood—except now it was gentle and reflective, conducive to building consensus about what we had dreamed up in those previous sessions. We went from the yellow quadrant—positive and energized—to the green—still positive, but now calm and rational.

Then we needed a third set of meetings, to sort out the nuts-and-bolts phase. In these sessions, we turned off the music. We sat quietly and addressed all of the details in a businesslike way and came up with timetables, budgets, contingency plans. We decided who would manage the research, who would oversee publicity, who would arrange for security and insurance. We went from the green to light blue in order to narrow our focus and engage in deductive reasoning. By the end of those sessions we had a workable, realistic plan for going forward.

Before the big conference began, we had one more decision to make: What was the feeling we hoped our audience members would take away? We wanted them to end up in the red quadrant—aware of the injustices in the status quo and motivated, even passionate, about making changes. Not merely enthusiastic, but a little angry, because anger is how we respond to unfairness. To manage that, we had to deliver closing remarks about our findings and the path forward in a way that activated our listeners. I didn't want the public officials to walk out saying, "Wow, that conference was a great experience!" I wanted them to realize that there was an emergency they needed to address. I wanted them energized with a sense of mission when they got back to work.

Now it's time to treat Regulation as a practical—necessary—skill we can master.

So far, we've been describing the RULER method as a fairly orderly procession from one step to the next, from Recognition to Understanding and so on. But human minds and emotions aren't so neatly organized, and we don't process information one piece at a time. Often, we regulate before we're even fully conscious of what we're feeling. Someone is rude to you at work, and your brain instantly jolts you from peaceful green into the fiery red quadrant of angry activation, ready to defend your dignity. Without thinking, you take a deep breath and get some distance. That's Regulation (specifically, implicit or automatic Regulation).

Emotion regulation can be as simple as this: You can't stand your neighbor? Avoid her. Your parents are coming to visit and you don't want them to see some of your more outré artwork? Hide it until they leave. You're tired? Splash some water on your face.

Emotion regulation is not about *not* feeling. Neither is it exerting tight control over what we feel. And it's not about banishing negative emotions and feeling only positive ones. Rather, emotion regulation starts with giving ourselves and others the permission to own our feelings—all of them.

Years ago, I visited a classroom in a high-poverty area of New York. A boy named George who was in the fourth grade shared that he was in the blue quadrant, and with good reasons: his pet hamster had been killed by a rat that morning. Later, I learned he lived in temporary housing, and his life was full of anxiety and uncertainty.

The teacher asked the class, "What can we do to support George today?" and the answers came back quickly. One student said, "Can I give you a hug?" Another said, "George, I'm here for you anytime today if you want to talk." The shift in George's facial expression was instant. He came to class distraught but was comforted by his peers in a way that let him know he was cared for. He wasn't being urged to shift out of the blue quadrant; rather, he was given support and affection so he could be comfortable where he was. George was no longer alone in his misery but now in the company of peers and a teacher who wanted to hear him and understand his needs. Too often we look for strategies that will shift people out of negative emotion spaces, but that's not always possible. During difficult times, sometimes we just need to be there for one another.

For the remainder of this chapter, we'll dive deeply into five broad categories of emotion regulation. Within each category, the number of specific strategies is virtually infinite, each one determined by the moment, context, and emotion, by our age, personality, and culture, by whatever came before and whatever we wish to happen next.

The first category is a strategy that literally keeps us alive: breathing. Specifically, *mindful breathing* helps us to calm the body and mind so we can be fully present and less reactive or overwhelmed by what's happening around us.

The second category we'll call *forward-looking strategies*. This simply means that we anticipate something will cause an unwanted emotion and either steer clear of it or modify our physical environment.

The third category is *attention-shifting strategies*. This takes many forms, but all are based on the same principle—that we can temper the impact of an emotion by diverting our attention away from its source. It can be as simple as turning on the TV, walking away from a stressful encounter, or repeating a positive phrase to ourselves.

The fourth we'll call *cognitive-reframing strategies*. We first analyze whatever's triggering an emotional experience and then find a new way of seeing it—essentially, transforming our perception of reality as a way of mastering it.

Finally, I'll introduce the *Meta-Moment*, a tool which helps us to act as our best selves would, as opposed to reacting (and overreacting) to emotional situations.

Mindful breathing

I'd like you to take two minutes to pause, get comfortable, and breathe naturally. If it will help, you can time yourself. Begin now.

How'd it go? Did you even do it? Or did you just keep reading? If you did try it, how did it feel? Did you get impatient, anxious, bored? Did your mind wander? Maybe it was the first time you've taken a minute for yourself all day, and you feel calm or centered. Allowing our minds to be idle is a major challenge for many of us given our busy lives. And it's especially hard when we're faced with strong emotions such as anxiety, anger, and even excitement.

Our brain responds to intense emotions by activating the sympathetic nervous system: our heart rate goes up, stress hormones and/or endorphins are released depending on the emotion, and (when pressured) we prepare to flee or freeze.

Mindful breathing helps us to hit the brake on the activation of our stress response system by decreasing our heart rate. Breathing through the nose is helpful because mouth breathing tends to be faster and shallower (think of a panting dog), which can reactivate the stress response system. And when we count our breaths or repeat a calming phrase while breathing, we regain balance and control because the area of the brain in charge shifts from the brain stem to the motor cortex. Breathing also helps us to reset the autonomic nervous system by activating the parasympathetic nervous system and inhibiting the sympathetic (excitatory) one.

When we breathe mindfully, we don't have to sit in a fancy yoga posture or use any special techniques. But it is important to have good posture whether sitting or standing. Mindful breathing can be practiced anywhere: at home, school, work, or even while trying to fall asleep.

It's best to build a practice of mindful breathing in small steps over time. Start by taking a few minutes a couple of times a week to sit and breathe mindfully. Over time you can build up to a five-, ten-, or even fifteen-minute practice each day. That way, when you are in the situation where you'll need to deactivate, you'll be prepared.

Do your best to

○ remove distractions such as your cell phone.
○ get comfortable.
○ close your eyes or lower your eyelids.
○ be aware of your posture and body. You can place your hand on a spot where you feel the breath, but it's not necessary.
○ breathe naturally.
  • You can count to 10: inhale 1/exhale 1, inhale 2/exhale 2, and so on until you get to 10. Then repeat.
  • Or you can breathe while repeating a phrase. I learned my favorite more than twenty years ago from Thich Nhat Hanh, a leader in the mindfulness community. It's simple: On the inhale you say "in" and on the exhale you say "out." Then "deep/slow," "calm/ease," "smile/release." Repeat. This particular one helps me at night when my mind is racing and I have a hard time falling asleep.
  • bring your attention back to your breath if you notice your mind wandering.

If you are like me and get easily distracted during the practice, you might start thinking: I can't do this. It's hopeless. Try to be an emotion scientist, not a judge about it. Even have a little self-compassion and try it again. You're exercising a new muscle. Once you're comfortable with these two basic exercises, you can try others, but it's not necessary. I've stuck with the basic ones for years.

Today, dozens of experiments demonstrate the benefits of mindful breathing on our emotional, social, and cognitive functioning. Over time, not only do we deactivate more quickly, but our ability to focus and to be present grows stronger. Research suggests that just fifteen minutes of this practice daily can positively affect our attunement to family and friends, emotional reactivity, attention, memory, immune function, hypertension, asthma, autonomic nervous system imbalances, and mental health.

Forward-looking strategies

The following strategies require enough self-awareness for us to know what exactly will set us off, or bring us joy, and why. We consider how we will feel in an upcoming situation and devise a plan ahead of time to alter the emotional impact. This skill depends on R, U, and L—Recognition, Understanding, and Labeling.

For instance, you have an aunt who always manages to infuriate you over Thanksgiving dinner. Rather than grit your teeth through another tense holiday, you decide in advance to sit at the opposite end of the table. Problem solved!

Or there's a subordinate at the office who's been after you for a one-on-one meeting, but there's a problem: he makes you nervous and you know it will be an extremely awkward session. You've been stalling him, but that only makes things worse, as your dread keeps growing. There's probably some good reason behind your aversion, but you can address that another day. Right now, a good regulation strategy would be to turn your one-on-one meeting into a group session with other employees on your team. The instant that solution occurs to you, you feel better.

This strategy requires some self-knowledge, but if we can predict which situations or encounters will provoke an emotional reaction, we can take measures to prevent them from happening.

When it's impossible to avert the future completely, we can still anticipate it and change it. Your annual job review is coming up, which always fills you with fear and insecurity for a week before it happens and outright dread as it finally takes place. But if you try to imagine every possible scenario—all the criticisms of your performance that your boss might bring up and all the calm, well-reasoned responses you will make in response—you might not be your usual stammering, defensive self when the time comes.

Likewise, avoidance is a strategy. It doesn't sound like an advisable one, but it can be useful under certain circumstances. I won't go to a certain restaurant because they have amazing fries and I can't resist them. So I stay away and save myself a lot of anguish. No great loss. You're in a store and the cashier is rude, but it's not as though you and he are likely to interact in the future, so there's no long-term need to do anything about it. Just never go near the place again or look for a different cashier.

However, if you realize that there have been other instances, at work or at home with your spouse or children, where you've just walked away from rudeness because you felt incapable of facing it down, and every time it happens you feel belittled and humiliated or enraged, maybe there's something else going on—like an inability to have a difficult conversation or stand up for yourself and deal with unpleasantness. Perhaps you need to find a long-term strategy better than avoidance.

There's another aspect of forward-looking strategies worth mastering. It involves pleasure only. Let's say you're having a hellish week at work, and you already know that Friday will be the absolute capper. You're dreading it, but if you schedule a date for Friday night or make plans to go to the beach as soon as you leave the office, you suddenly have something great waiting for you at the end of the tunnel. Or if you have a root canal appointment looming, you can plan to do something you love right afterward and give yourself a treat to look forward to. As a rule, doing something you enjoy is a very effective strategy for regulating negative emotions.

Attention-shifting strategies

These take many forms, but all are based on the same principle—that we can temper the impact of an emotion by diverting our attention from it. It can be as simple as looking away from a stressful encounter or as reflective as delivering a self-talk as though we were speaking to a friend who was under duress, telling them to visualize being on a beautiful beach.

Bored waiting in a cashier line, so you check your Instagram feed? That's distraction. Pretty common today. Not terribly useful. You could have devoted those moments to thinking about a new business idea you had or planning your vacation. Still, it beats standing there and steaming.

Or your credit card payment is due tomorrow and your checking account balance is low, so you ease the angst by vowing to change your spending habits and start saving. If it makes you feel better, fine. It's a good way to avert moments like this in the future. But diverting your attention won't pay the bill that's staring you in the face.

A nervous wreck until you get back the results from a blood test, so you binge-watch Netflix? Better than suffering. So frustrated over your inability to lose weight that only ice cream will ease the pain? Could help you through the next fifteen minutes, but maybe not the perfect strategy going forward for achieving that particular goal.

The list of potential distractions is infinite. Everything from day-dreaming to drugs. Food—snacking—is a great short-term strategy, not unlike other recreational mood enhancers for its ability to provide physical comfort that overrides mental anxiety. It's that surge of sugar in the bloodstream that prompts the rush of pleasure to the brain. If you depend on junk food as a regulation strategy just occasionally, you're like the rest of us. If it's three times a day, you may have some emotional *and* physical issues to deal with.

It's possible to distract ourselves to such a degree that we avoid deal-ing with anything difficult—even when our lives would be improved by facing reality and doing something about it. What we commonly call "denial" is just an extreme form of distraction—akin to burying our heads in the sand during a crisis.

Still, it's emotion regulation.

Procrastination is a popular way of creating some emotional distance using time rather than space. If a situation is causing you stress, just decide you'll deal with it next week, or next month, or at some indefinite point in the future. Poof, it's gone. Politicians and public officials love this one—in their world it's known as "kicking the can down the road," and it allows them to avoid dealing with painful deficits, deadlines, and other challenges. Procrastination must be effective, otherwise we wouldn't make such abundant use of it. But like other cheap, easy fixes, it's got plenty of potential to harm and not much to help.

"Self-talk" is something we all do at one time or another—it's simply expressing our thoughts silently as though we're speaking to ourselves out loud. The best part about self-talk is that it's effortless, since we all talk to ourselves from time to time. Many of us aren't particularly nice about it—think of when you've called yourself an idiot if something goes wrong. Positive self-talk just requires us to be kind and empathic when we do it. The challenge, as we've learned, at least in Western cultures, is that our inborn negativity bias contributes to our negative self-talk, not to mention all of the negative talk we've picked up from our parents and peers. We can't just drop it—we need to replace it. Harsh self-criticism activates the sympathetic nervous system (fight/flight) and elevates stress hormones. Self-compassion, on the other hand, triggers the mammalian caregiving system and hormones of affiliation and love such as oxytocin.

Researchers Ethan Kross at the University of Michigan and Jason Moser at Michigan State University have studied how our brains respond to self-talk. In particular, they compared what happens when we address ourselves in the third person rather than the first, meaning that I'd start by saying, "Marc . . . ," as though I were speaking to someone other than myself. It may not seem like much of a difference, but it turns out to be significant.

In one experiment, subjects were shown neutral and disturbing images or asked to recall negative moments from their own lives. By monitoring their emotional brain activity, the researchers found that the subjects' distress decreased rapidly—within one second—when they performed self-talk in the third person compared with the first person.

Why would that make a difference? Jason Moser wrote, "Essentially, we think referring to yourself in the third person leads people to think about themselves more similarly to how they think about others, and you can see evidence for this in the brain. That helps people gain a tiny bit of psychological distance from their experiences, which can often be useful for regulating emotions." Essentially, third-person self-talk is a way of being empathetic to ourselves.

I find myself making use of self-talk to regulate my own moods all the time. I have found it very useful to have go-to phrases for different purposes. When I start catastrophizing, I say, "Marc, you are making this up." When I'm overwhelmed before bed, I say, "Marc, you know this feeling is impermanent. Go to bed. You'll be fine in the morning."

Sometimes, self-talk is more elaborate. I give seminars before groups all around the world. Most of the time, I'm energetic and enthusiastic about my mission and the people who want to learn about it. Sometimes, though, it's the third talk I've given in the past two days, and it's coming at the end of a long work session, and all I really want to do is lie down in my hotel room and watch HBO. Instead, I've got to get up and perform for the next three hours.

Here's what I tell myself:

"Marc, you're about to talk with one hundred school superintendents. They oversee tens of thousands of teachers, each of whom is in front of classrooms all day long, educating hundreds of thousands of children. And you now have the opportunity to share something that could have a profound effect on the lives of those kids. What happens tonight in that room will help those children to learn better and succeed not only in school but in *life*."

"Wow!" I reply. "How lucky am I to be in this position?" And with that I'm psyched and ready to go.

Cognitive-reframing strategies

"There is nothing either good or bad, but thinking makes it so," says Hamlet. That idea is the basis for our fourth, most sophisticated, intellectually engaged method of emotion regulation—*cognitive-reframing strategies*, better known in the research literature as *reappraisal*.

In a sense, this can be seen as an offshoot of cognitive behavioral therapy, in which people are encouraged to seek alternate ways of viewing their difficulties as a path to coming into balance with them.

For our purposes, we use reappraisal as a way to reimagine or reframe whatever is triggering an emotional experience and then react instead to that new interpretation.

Here's an example. You come down to breakfast, say good morning to your partner, and are met with a surly look instead of the usual warm greeting. If your first reaction is that you did nothing to deserve such rudeness, you may hold a grudge all day (or at least until dinner). You may even respond in kind, which will only perpetuate the foul mood in the air.

Instead, you could pause and consider alternate reasons for what just happened. Maybe she's anxious about something she's afraid to talk to you about? Perhaps he's furious about a work interaction that had nothing to do with you but has left him humiliated and hurt? Those possibilities might remind you that she or he is never this rude under normal circumstances, and suddenly you're feeling empathetic and wondering how you can help. And in that fashion, your emotional response has been regulated, to the benefit of all.

The basic principles of reframing are that we consciously choose to view a situation in a way that generates the least negative emotion in us or we attempt to take the perspective of the person who is activating you and assume the best intention. For example, if a clerk is rude and dismissive, we could think, This guy is being a jerk to me, or, He obviously has a real problem with women, or, Maybe he thinks I don't have enough money to shop here—all of which would make you at least indirectly responsible for his behavior. With reframing, we might think instead, This guy must *really* hate his job, or, I wonder if he's just gotten bad news—both of which might turn your bruised ego into feelings of compassion or even curiosity.

The goal of reframing isn't only to regulate bruised feelings. You could be a teacher on your first day at a new school and the faculty meeting leaves you crestfallen—the teachers all seem so inexperienced and ill prepared. Instead of despairing, you could view this as a chance to mentor younger colleagues and have an impact on the entire school and come away excited instead of depressed.

Here's an example from an experiment conducted with employees at a large financial institution. Over the course of a week, one group of workers was shown videos about the harmful effects of stress—bad for health, detrimental to job performance, an obstacle to learning and growth. A second group of workers saw videos containing the opposite message—that stress is actually good for our health, inspiring better job performance as well as learning and growth.

Participants who watched the three-minute "stress is positive" videos three times a week had a significant reduction in negative health symptoms and an increase in work performance compared with those who watched the "stress is negative" videos. Other studies show that people who endorse the stress-is-enhancing mindset have a stronger desire to receive feedback.

Research done at Harvard found similar results. Students who were asked to think of pretest anxiety as being beneficial performed better on exams than a control group. In another experiment, reframing anxiety as excitement was found to improve negotiating and public-speaking skills.

Studies conducted using functional fMRI measures of brain activation found that reappraisal significantly dampens activity in the amygdala, an area of our brain that becomes activated when we experience strong emotions, and instead activates the lateral temporal cortical areas of the brain, which help us to modulate our emotional responses.

As is true of all regulation strategies, reframing has the potential to harm as well as help.

Imagine: You're at a party when your spouse shares something that embarrasses you. You're about to blow your top and storm out of the room, but instead you resist the urge, take a series of mindful breaths, and reconsider what just happened.

"He didn't *mean* to humiliate me," you tell yourself. That might help—at least now you believe he didn't intentionally hold you up to ridicule.

"He had a couple drinks too many," you reason. That could also lessen the sting. Now the martinis are at fault.

"I'm being hypersensitive, it wasn't such a big deal," you decide. And that's possible—maybe you're just tired and feeling more fragile than usual. Perhaps you're the only one in the room who thinks what he said was inappropriate.

Reframing the incident calmed you down and prevented an ugly scene, so we can consider this a successful regulation of a very strong emotion.

Or not.

Same scenario. You conduct the same self-talk to help you handle the situation without melting down. Until you recall that it's the third time something like this has happened in the past two months. And deep down you believe that maybe his intentions weren't so pure and he took some satisfaction from everyone having a laugh at your expense. And he's been having a few too many drinks a little too often lately. Now you realize that you weren't being hypersensitive—any normal person would have been outraged by what he said in the middle of a crowded party.

Which means that reframing has been allowing you to live in denial or disavowal about something unspoken and unhealthy that's going on between the two of you. He's attacking you in a passive-aggressive way, and for some reason you're allowing it. You haven't called him on it, and you haven't even admitted to yourself how bad it makes you feel. Your reluctance is understandable—once you face your feelings, you'll have to do something about them. It may not be easy. But until you do, and start dealing with them instead of regulating them out of existence, things won't get any better.

And that's how it can sometimes go with cognitive reappraisal, a very intelligent and helpful—and persuasive—strategy for emotion regulation.

When it comes to reappraisal, we need to ask ourselves: Am I doing this simply to justify avoiding a difficult, sensitive problem? Am I doing this because I know that addressing the issue is going to lead to a long, tortured, anguished conversation? In that case, reappraisal may be a useful short-term solution—you're on your way to a party, not the ideal moment for an ugly face-off. But it's also a poor long-term strategy, because ducking the issue now will only ensure that it will reemerge later on.

This is why we must make the effort to be an emotion scientist—we need to check in with ourselves regularly, to evaluate our feelings honestly, without judging ourselves for having them. Every time we believe we've successfully employed a strategy to regulate our feelings, we have to ask: That may have worked (for now), but what did it accomplish (for the long run)?

The Meta-Moment

Here we are, finally, at the pinnacle of emotion regulation, the most complex and also the most potentially rewarding of the RULER skills. But there's a catch.

As we all know, our best attempts at calm, thoughtful reflection work only when we feel in control of our emotions. If you're raging with resentment or crushed by disappointment, it's unlikely that you're capable of the extended reasoning required to see a situation in a new light. In that scenario, you'd first need to bring down your emotional temperature, to lower your activation and give yourself the space required for rational thought. Maybe you take a few deep breaths, a few steps back, a walk around the block.

Then, maybe you're ready for the Meta-Moment.

A decade ago, Robin Stern, psychoanalyst and associate director of our center, and I were wondering why, as a society, so many people are addicted to strategies that derail them from achieving their goals. Robin had worked with hundreds of patients who were unsuccessful even after learning strategies, and I observed schoolchildren and educators who didn't employ the strategies they were learning, even when they knew they were helpful.

Many of us were exposed to destructive strategies starting early in life—negative talk, screaming, blaming, and so on. Those responses require little cognitive control but are often effective at getting rid of negative feelings and providing (temporary) gratification. In the moment, we fail to realize that these strategies also can ruin our relationships. They fail to take in long-term consequences and derail us from achieving our goals.

We needed to suggest something—a tool—that would help people find beneficial strategies on their own.

So we developed a tool we call the Meta-Moment. In simplest terms, it's a pause. The Meta-Moment involves hitting the brakes and stepping out of time. We call it *meta* because it's a moment about a moment. We often associate it with counting, as in "one, two, three," or even one to ten, depending on the severity of the emotion we're struggling to manage. Taking one or more deep breaths may also be a part of it. Anything to give ourselves a little room to maneuver and deactivate.

This is where we stop the action and say, "Am I hearing this correctly?" Or even, "I need to pause and take a deep breath right now so I don't blow my top, break down sobbing, or react in some other way I will probably regret." Looking at the encounter dispassionately may help us go beyond our first impulse and find a better response. As the author and consultant Justin Bariso wrote, "Pausing helps you refrain from making a permanent decision based on a temporary emotion."

Instinctively, we sense that this will help, and biology proves us right. Pausing and taking a deep breath activates the parasympathetic nervous system, which reduces the release of cortisol, a major stress hormone, and naturally lowers our emotional temperature.

Pausing also gives us the chance to quickly ask a few questions that might be useful, such as "How have I handled situations like this in the past?" Or "What would my *best self* do right now?" That ideal, hypothetical person comprises attributes we would use to describe our best selves from our own perspective and from the perspective of others—how we'd like to be seen and experienced. For some people it's a set of adjectives such as compassionate, intelligent, or conscientious; for others it can be an image or an object. A good friend who is principal of a middle school has a Smurf on her desk that reminds her to be her best self.

Visualizing our best self redirects our attention away from the "trigger" and toward our values. This helps us to choose a helpful regulation strategy such as positive self-talk or reappraisal and then respond accordingly.

A couple of years ago, I had a student who raised his hand in class and said, "I have a question that I don't think *even you'll know* how to answer." To say that I was activated is an understatement; arrogance is a trigger for me. I wanted to reply: I might not know the answer, but remember I grade your papers. I would have thrown in a few expletives too. Instead, I reached down into my "professor of emotional intelligence" self and said, "How about if I get questions from some of the other students now and we can chat after class?" There, I politely informed him that his question could have been worded more diplomatically.

More recently, I was giving a presentation to a large group when someone challenged me on a point I was making. She didn't just ask a question or offer a dissenting opinion. She came at me with the intention of putting me down. "A lot of us in the room would not necessarily agree with that model," she said. My first impulse was to fire right back and embarrass her in front of her colleagues with a comment like "A lot of us, meaning you and your thirty personalities." But I didn't allow myself that petty pleasure. Instead, I took myself out of the moment, visualized my best self as "the feelings master," and paused as though I were formulating a reply. In that small window of time I calmed myself, then made a comment without belittling her and moved on. "I'd love to connect with you later to hear your thoughts," I said. Nobody in that room knew how close I came to losing it. Truth is, a couple of years prior, I likely would have crumbled.

The Meta-Moment is not just for down-regulating unpleasant emotions. Sometimes our best selves help us to stand up for what's right. Once, during a speech, a colleague bullied me in an unusual way—he joked about the fact that I was bullied as a child. I hate to admit it, but my first impulse was to run onstage and deliver a flying dropkick to his head. I regressed to feeling like that middle schooler being pushed around in the locker room. But I took a Meta-Moment and waited until after the presentation, when I went up to him and said, "I have no idea what motivated you to say those words, but it wasn't cool and you can't ever do it again."

I count these as victories for the Meta-Moment.

How skilled are you at taking a Meta-Moment? What adjectives characterize your best self? What are your go-to strategies when you are triggered or caught off guard? Do you ignore your feelings, act out, or meet them head-on?

When your boss criticizes your work and you feel disappointed, devastated, or resentful, how successful are you at taking a Meta-Moment, then saying to yourself something like "Feedback is a gift, there is always something I can learn."

When your daughter won't do her homework, do you argue, threaten, plead, grimace in disgust, explode in rage . . . or do you take a deep breath, evoke your best self, think about the most effective strategy with this particular child, and calmly take action?

Here are the steps to take so you can begin practicing the Meta-Moment.

1. *Sense the shift:* You are activated, caught off guard, or have an impulse to say or do something that you might regret. There is a shift in your thinking or physiology or both.
2. *Stop or pause!* Create the space before you respond. Step back and breathe. Breathe again.
3. *See your best self.* You imagine your best self. You think of adjectives or even an image that helps your *best self* appear in vivid detail. You might also think about your reputation: how do you want to be seen, talked about, and experienced? What would you do if someone you respect were watching?
4. *Strategize* and *act.* You reach into your RULER tool kit (for instance, positive self-talk or reframing) and choose the path that will support you in closing the gap between your "triggered" self and your emerging best self. (Always the last step.)

There are a few, final aspects of Regulation we need to consider. Because emotion regulation requires brainpower—moving from automatic and unhelpful to deliberate and helpful strategies is hard work!—it depends on seemingly unrelated factors such as diet, exercise, and sleep. When we eat poorly, our minds don't function properly. Too much sugar or refined grain causes our blood glucose to spike and then plummet, which affects cognitive functioning and self-control, especially around healthy eating. Easy solution: Make sure you have some healthy snacks in your desk at work or set a reminder on your phone to ensure you nibble every three hours or so.

Too little physical activity has a negative effect on our mental capacity and moods. In one study, subjects were exposed to a stressor, and then half of the participants did aerobic exercise while the others did not. The exercisers reported feeling significantly less negative than the other group. Even anxiety and depression can be reduced by exercise. Accumulating research is showing how a regular yoga practice might be beneficial for both our mental and physical health.

Poor quality or insufficient sleep has similar effects on our emotions—when we're tired, our defenses are down and our ability to function mentally is low. Sleep serves a restorative function. When we don't get enough, or we get too much, we show more symptoms of anxiety and depression, greater fatigue, and hostility. Inadequate sleep is associated with reduced connections between brain regions responsible for cognitive control and behavior and the use of effective emotion regulation strategies.

There are two more measures we can take to safeguard our overall well-being. The first is by doing things we love. Spend time with family and friends, pursue passions and pastimes, get in touch with your spiritual side, immerse yourself in nature, read a good book, watch a funny movie. We build up cognitive reserves that way, which will help us when emotional turmoil inevitably strikes. We are hardwired to seek social contact and support—people who lack it are prone to anxiety, depression, and cardiovascular disease.

The second measure is to practice mindful breathing, which is perhaps the ultimate prevention strategy. As we've learned, daily practice enhances our ability to be present, accept feelings as they come and go, and not be overly reactive or overwhelmed by them.

Just take everything we know about how to maintain good physical and mental health and apply it to your emotional fitness. It's all connected.

With that, we've completed our education in the final RULER skill. But we're not quite finished yet.

Learning the five RULER skills and how and why they work is essential. But it's just the beginning of your education. Now comes the part where you put them all to good use.

It's not so simple, learning five interrelated skills all at once. Think of what it was like to learn any skill you now possess. For example, it took me four years of daily practice to get a black belt and another ten years to obtain a fifth-degree black belt. Like learning a martial art, developing emotion skills takes time. It takes work. It takes practice. It takes openness to feedback. It takes refinement.

Owing to the emotional nature of these particular skills, you may find that you're better at some than at others. It's certainly that way for me. I know that I'm often better at R, U, and L than I am at E or R. I suppose that means I'm better at the thinking parts of RULER than I am at putting them into action. Recently, after a long, exhausting day of delayed flights, missed connections, and other irritations, I felt that I was on the verge of a meltdown. Then I asked myself, If a college professor with a doctorate in psychology has difficulty regulating emotions, what must it be like for a nine-year-old child or an adult under genuinely challenging pressures who have had little to no training in emotion skills? That calmed me down in a hurry. It also reminded me how much work needs to be done to ensure every child gets an emotion education.

I think Mike Tyson had it right when he said, "Everybody has a plan until they get punched in the mouth." What's true in the boxing ring is true everywhere else—it's easy to say that from now on we'll master all our emotional responses, until our significant other or cranky child or unreasonable boss triggers us with a word or a look, and suddenly all the RULER training goes out the window.

So, along with permission to feel, we must also give ourselves permission to fail. When that happens, we can only try again—take a deep breath or two, envision our best selves, and start over at the first R. At such moments, we also need the courage to apologize and to forgive ourselves as we'd forgive others. Courage can even mean seeking professional help when all else fails.

We'll never stop having to work at being our best selves. But the payoff is worth it: better health, decision making, relationships, better everything.

Of course, all the emotion mastery in the world won't help much if everyone else is still playing by the bad old rules of engagement. As Uncle Marvin and I discovered decades ago, it's not enough to teach these skills to schoolchildren. Their teachers must also become emotion scientists. And their parents too. And everyone else with any influence over their lives, including employers and work colleagues. Which is what the next section is all about.

PART THREE

APPLYING EMOTION SKILLS FOR OPTIMUM WELL-BEING AND SUCCESS

9

Emotions at Home

A WOMAN APPROACHED ME after a seminar I did for parents and caregivers. She whispered, "Can we talk privately? I am really worried about my son."

"Sure," I said, "tell me the problem."

"I am afraid he has no emotional intelligence," she said. "He's throwing things and is just too aggressive. He's different from my oldest son, who is gregarious and highly skilled. I am really worried. My husband and I are a mess. Should we bring him to a psychologist?"

I made some suggestions for how she could support her child in learning how to regulate emotions, but she said, "We can't use any of those strategies."

"Why not?" I asked.

"Because he's only eleven months old."

I stood there speechless. The first thing that came to mind to say was, "Yes, I think you should call a psychologist—for *you*." Instead, I took a breath and gently suggested that maybe she was being overly worried about her son's emotional intelligence and could wait a little while longer before seeking professional help.

We all arrive in this world programmed differently where emotions are concerned. Each of us has a different threshold for being provoked, activated, aroused, startled. Some of us experience feelings more intensely than others. We recover from emotional reactions at different speeds. But these individual differences don't determine whether we will develop emotion skills. Research shows that even highly reactive kids who are raised in nurturing families can turn out just fine.

Of course we're all concerned about the emotional lives of our children. We know what's at stake—virtually everything. As we've seen already, their physical and mental well-being, their ability to learn in school, their future success at work and in families of their own, all depend on it. There's no greater measure of how we did as parents than the success of our kids in this regard. Few influences can match those of family and home.

But *which* home?

There's the home where we grew up, where our emotional lives were formed. We're not born with emotion knowledge; we mostly respond to stimuli—we're hungry, we're cold, we're uncomfortable for one reason or another, and so we react. Nature provides that response to make sure we get the attention we need to survive infancy. Everything beyond that is learned in the nest.

Along the way, as we learn what we need to be an adult and to sustain a home or family, we take in the emotional experiences, like the air we breathe. We carry those emotional patterns forward with us—the good and the bad—often replicating them. And in our new home, the cycle repeats—built on the emotional foundations of the one where we started out.

Many of us go through life trying our hardest to avoid precisely that fate. We strive to be anything *but* our parents. And then, inevitably, comes the moment when we hear ourselves say, "Where did that come from?" Suddenly we realize we've been carrying our parents around inside us all our lives.

When there are two adults building a family, there are even more emotional inheritances in that home. And even if there are no children present—or you live alone—that past is always somewhere inside of you.

Given this, what steps can we take to create healthy home environments, places where our children and loved ones will feel supported, valued, treasured, understood, *heard*? Homes filled with patience and acceptance and humor and joy?

Few parents today would argue with the idea that their children will do best if they're well loved. That wasn't always so. Early in the twentieth century, the fields of child psychology and development were divided over how best to raise children, especially on the merits of strictness or leniency, discipline or tenderness. The president of the American Psychological Association, John B. Watson, warned in 1915 that too much love and comforting was dangerous for children and that their lives would be spoiled by cuddling.

Today, nothing could sound more misguided or damaging. Current scientific research on attachment of children to parents, on the power of feeling seen and felt, and on the benefits of comfort all show one thing: Children do best with demonstrative love and caring.

But parents seem ambivalent when it comes to their children's emotional lives. I routinely encounter RULER-resistant parents who think I'm advocating for everybody sitting in a circle on the living room floor and *discussing their feelings* ad nauseam. They see our work as overindulging their children instead of preparing them for real life.

What those parents miss is that a focus on emotion skills is about real, practical *skills*.

Permission to feel doesn't mean obsessing over every time somebody is mean to us or ignores us. It's really just the opposite—teaching the ability to get through those moments, to learn from them, and to continue to function normally. Emotion skills are a bulwark against the epidemic of anger, bullying, disengagement, anxiety, and dread in this country, especially among young people. They clear away the most persistent drags on our creativity, relationships, decisions, and health.

Permission to feel *strengthens*. It's not always easy to face the truth about who we are and to reckon with our own and our children's emotional lives. But it is a whole lot better than the alternative: denial, overreacting, and so on. You teach your children to express their emotions by skillfully expressing yours. Conversely, if you are reluctant to express your feelings, or do so only sparingly, in as few words as possible, then that's what your children will learn to do when they grow up. This is why we adults need to be open to learning and practicing strategies in our own emotional lives before we can support our kids.

Researchers have found many ways that parents' own emotions affect their children's:

Beliefs about feelings. Family researchers such as John Gottman and developmental psychologists such as Amy Halberstadt have shown that parents who value emotions tend to be aware of their children's feelings and are able to act like coaches. They don't respond with threats of discipline when their kids express anger or sadness—instead, they see strong feelings as a central part of healthy development. Parents who view emotions as harmful or disruptive are the ones who command their children to "suck it up" and see their kids' emotional expressions as manipulative. Those are the same parents who mask their own emotions and send implicit messages that feelings are unimportant.

Even when we do acknowledge others' emotions, we have to be careful about *how* we do so. Boys and girls often receive different messages about emotions from parents. And these gender differences tend to increase with age: Nancy Eisenberg, a professor of developmental psychology at Arizona State University, reported that there are few gender differences in preschool children, but by second grade larger disparities emerge. For example:

- Mothers speak more to daughters about feelings and display a wider range of feelings to daughters than to sons.
- Fathers discourage boys from expressing emotional vulnerability and use tougher language with sons than they do with daughters.
- When parents tell stories to their preschool children, they use more emotion words with daughters than with sons.
- Mothers smile more and are more expressive to infant and toddler girls than boys and talk more about sadness with daughters and more about anger with sons.

Emotion vocabulary. Most of us are unaware of how important vocabulary is to emotion skills. As we've seen, using many different words implies valuable distinctions—that we're not always simply angry but are sometimes annoyed, irritated, frustrated, disgusted, aggravated, and so on. If we can't discern the difference, it suggests that we can't understand it either. It's the difference between a rich emotional life and an impoverished one. Your child will inherit the one you provide.

In one study, researchers found that mothers who used more sophisticated language when talking about feelings had children who were better at regulating their own emotions. The authors wrote, "The ability to talk about one's own affective state has its most obvious importance for regulating affect in its power to enlist others as sources of aid or comfort." What that means, essentially, is that if mothers and fathers use many words to describe emotions rather than just a few basic ones, their children will be better able to express their feelings to others. They'll also be more empathic.

Co-regulation. Researchers use the term *co-regulation* to refer to how we affect one another's feelings, moving another's feelings up or down by our own actions. In the parent-child dyad, the child is an active participant in his or her own regulation, but the parent is the source of the strategy.

At the most basic level, it includes a caregiver's warmth, responsiveness, and sensitivity, as well as methods for buffering a child against stress and creating routines to promote a sense of security. For young children it might include offering strategies such as distraction: "You sound upset. Are you angry because he took your toy? Let's play with this toy together instead."

Another way involves scaffolding children's self-regulation of emotion using prompts: "What happened? How are you feeling? How do you want to feel?" The adult may act as a partner to support problem solving—"Why don't you let him play with your toy? After two minutes, I'll make sure he gives it back"—and reappraisal: "Perhaps he thought it was his own toy and not yours. I see he has a very similar one behind him."

And yet another strategy is metacognitive prompting, which emphasizes empowering children to generate and/or choose from alternative emotion regulation strategies: "Is there another way to think about what happened? What could you do instead? What's worked before when you've felt this way?"

I'm an obsessive eavesdropper on families in public. For me, it's research. Sometimes I find skilled parents who nurture their children's developing emotion skills. But not always.

This happened one morning while I was eating breakfast in a hotel restaurant:

"You're going to calm down right *now*," the father said to his daughter, who looked to be about three years old. "Thank you for ruining our day." I couldn't tell what prompted his outburst.

He then picked up the menu, ordered breakfast, and turned to his phone, as did the little girl's mother. For thirty minutes, that man never once looked up at his daughter or his wife. As they rose to leave, he turned at last to his daughter and said, "You're not going to behave that way again, are you?"

It wasn't a question.

"If you continue to behave like this, you aren't going swimming for the rest of the vacation."

The child began to sob. Do you think she cried because she couldn't go swimming? If you asked that three-year-old child how she was feeling—if she had adult language—you'd probably hear that she felt ignored, stifled, worthless in her father's eyes.

This father lacked the ability to recognize, understand, and label his daughter's feelings, and it broke my heart. As the family left the restaurant, I wondered: Was this a typical morning for them? Does this little girl believe she has the permission to feel? What is the implicit message her dad is sending her about her character? What learning will she carry forward into her future? How would a RULER-ized father manage the situation?

On a train once, I watched a mother and her son, who looked to be about seven. I first noticed them when I heard her say to the boy, "Remember, *train behavior.*" When I looked up I saw that she was staring at her cell phone and he was standing next to the seat. Two minutes later, he was wandering down the aisle. "I need you to *sit,*" she said. He did, and she went back to her phone. A few minutes later he was up again, walking around, until she noticed and said, *"Remember your train behavior!"* This little comedy kept playing out, and I was riveted. Finally, when he jumped up again, she screamed, *"Sit! And look at me when I'm talking to you!"* This was accompanied by a finger pointing to the seat next to hers and a piercing glare into his eyes.

I remember thinking, I have to put up with an hour of this? I wondered what would happen if I went over to her and said, "Excuse me, ma'am, but I am the director of the Yale Center for Emotional Intelligence, and I'd like to give you a little advice about how to handle this situation better."

What I really wanted to do was go to her son and whisper, "Quick, run away now while you can!"

Sometimes parents avoid dealing with their child's feelings by turning to technology as a way of removing themselves from the stress of the moment. According to research, this only increases the child's misery and inspires even more bad behavior . . . which parents then use as an excuse to isolate themselves even further. Children feel unimportant when parents use electronic devices during meals or conversations. Toddlers express more distress particularly when their mothers use their phones. And parents who are engrossed in their devices while at restaurants respond most harshly when their children want attention.

What about children's use of technology? According to a 2018 report by the Pew Research Center, 45 percent of teenagers are online "almost constantly" and U.S. high school seniors spend about six hours a day texting, on social media sites, or surfing the Internet. Research conducted by Jean Twenge, a professor at San Diego State University, shows that more hours of screen time are associated with lower well-being in children and adolescents; that higher users show less curiosity, self-control, and emotional stability; and that twice as many high versus low users of screens are diagnosed with anxiety or depression.

Okay, now it's time to examine how we were raised and search our memories for clues about the family we carry in our heads.

Take a moment and think back to the home you grew up in. Consider how it felt to be in your home, your relationship with your mom, dad, or caregiver. With that in mind, what's one word you would use to describe the emotional climate of your childhood home?

Here's a summary of thousands of responses from people across the globe. They fall into three categories: about 70 percent of the terms were negative, 20 percent were positive, and 10 percent were neutral.

The top negative responses: stuck, heavy, toxic, suppressed, inconvenient, stunted, avoidant, blind, intense, and unsupportive.

The top positive answers: supportive, loving, caring, nurturing, and accepting.

The top neutral words: unaware, selective, clueless, even, and neutral.

When I asked my brother this question, he immediately wrote back, "Ashtrays, hangers, and belts!" I knew exactly what he meant.

Ask yourself these questions: What did you learn about emotions growing up? What did you witness? Which feelings did your parents easily express, and which were never displayed? How did your parents handle your emotions, especially the difficult ones such as anger, fear, sadness? Were they emotion scientists, trying to figure out what you were feeling and why, as a way of helping you to deal with it? Or were they judges, blaming or finding fault with you for how you felt? Did you feel free to say what you felt? Did your parents' behavior encourage you to express, or did they send an implicit message to suppress your emotions?

Another way to think about this is to consider any defining moments—key points in your childhood that influenced who you are today. They can be memories of people or events that stand out as having a positive or negative effect on your development. Maybe these took place at home, or school, or the playground. What are some of your key defining moments?

Really think about this—try to remember what it was like in your home, at your school, with your family and friends. What were the positives that make you smile to recall? What were the painful or stressful moments, perhaps ones you've spent your life trying hard to forget? They matter just like the happy ones—no more but no less. Now, see what connections, if any, you can make between those moments, good and bad, and the adult you are today and the emotional life of your family.

Given our natural bias to remember negative events better than positive ones, I often think back to the bullying and abuse I suffered in elementary and middle school. One of my strongest memories of my childhood was when my parents made me run around the block on Christmas Eve before they would let me open presents. (Somehow, they believed that was an effective strategy to help me to lose weight.) But

I also had other, happy experiences, such as studying martial arts and earning my black belt, my girlfriend and best friend from high school, spending time with Uncle Marvin. Those were great times that brought me joy. Ultimately, it was both the positive and the negative experiences that led me to dedicate my life to helping others find the permission to feel and to express what they're feeling without shame or fear.

Once we've acknowledged the power of the past in our current emotional lives, we're ready to begin dealing with the present. RULER shows us how: First we recognize what we're feeling, so that we may understand why. Only then can we see *how* our feelings drive us to act—meaning what triggers us. We can regulate our emotional responses only if we can anticipate what will set us off.

When I ask parents to name their triggers, I get quick answers. Nobody has to think long before compiling this list:

"I'm triggered every day at seven forty A.M., when the war over getting my child up and dressed and out of the house on time begins."

"When I have to repeat the same thing over and over."

"When I've gone to all the trouble of cooking dinner and they refuse to eat."

"That snotty tone of voice no matter what I ask."

"Her bedroom is a pigsty."

"The never-ending arguing and fighting."

"Any time I'm reminded that we've raised two spoiled, entitled brats."

If you're a parent or caregiver, what are your triggers? What can you add to this list?

Once we air out that list of grievances, I ask parents how they typically respond to being triggered. These answers don't come so quickly. It takes a certain amount of honesty and bravery to confess how fierce and disproportionate our reactions can be:

"I scream at my daughter—*scream*. At the top of my lungs."

"I threaten."

"I'll take things away."

"I give the silent treatment."

"I've guilted them into doing what I wanted them to do."

"I blame my wife for not controlling them."

"I've bribed them to behave."

One mother told this story: Her high school son's sleepaway camp didn't work out one summer, so he returned home. "And he was slowly driving me out of my mind. He was a slob. He made the house a mess. He refused to look for work. So, he was always there. It got to the point where I couldn't even look at him, I was so irritated and frustrated. When I got to the breaking point I would lock myself in the bathroom. After about a month of that, my husband asked me if I had a urinary tract infection."

Do any of these reactions look familiar to you? What are your automatic, go-to strategies when you are triggered? When we feel threatened by our kids, our compassion switch turns off.

When I tell audiences how extreme reactions, over the course of time, can actually alter the brain structure of their children, the room goes quiet. Everyone is silently totaling up the times they lost their temper and went crazy on their kids, sizing up how much permanent damage they did to those impressionable young minds. The mood turns serious. Parents are mortified and filled with regret.

"It's pretty scary to think that all the yelling and screaming I've been doing for the past six years has damaged my kids' brains forever," one mother said, speaking for everyone in the room.

"Well," I tell them, "you don't have to worry too much, because a child's brain is still plastic, meaning that the structure is always changing. The minute you start regulating your emotions better, their brains will change to reflect that."

There's a sigh of relief all across the room.

"However," I say. "This doesn't get you off the hook. It doesn't mean you can keep yelling and screaming and punishing and stressing everybody out. It just means that if you can start regulating your emotions now, and help your children to regulate theirs, then there's hope."

"Triggered" is a telling word choice to describe the way we react to our emotions. We say it as though there's something outside us pulling a trigger—your child talked back in a rude tone, or stomped her foot, and that's what triggered your anger. But the trigger is inside us, not out there. We have to take responsibility for our actions rather than shift the blame elsewhere. It may not have felt like a choice, but it surely was—we decide how we'll respond to life's provocations. Don't want to explode in rage every time that kid is disrespectful? Come up with a better way to respond. Clearly, the old way—matching nastiness for nastiness—wasn't working.

So, what does work? This brings us back to the final R of RULER—Regulation, of our own emotional responses and those of our children too. The first step of Regulation, the single most powerful force in our arsenal, is the Meta-Moment. The pause for a breath (or two) when we're about to react in a way we'd really rather avoid.

Pausing to breathe when challenged is an ancient technique for mastering our responses to life. But that's just where the emotion regulation process begins. A breath can deactivate a strong reaction and buy us a second or two to think. But the full Meta-Moment is key.

Okay, so we've inhaled and exhaled deeply and hit the pause button. We covered this in chapter 8. Now what?

Something we call your *best self*.

By that we mean the ideal parent, the one who is kind, loving, patient, nurturing, calm, fair, reasonable, supportive, and encouraging. The same parent who never acts irrationally out of anger or frustration, who is never sarcastic, seething, withering, dictatorial, or scary.

Sounds like most parents, right? I wish. Never going to happen. We're all far too human and fallible for that. But the best self is like a golden ideal we can hold in our heads. We may not be that best self all of the time. We may not even get very close most of the time. But it's important to know *that* person well. It's the one you aspire to be. If during the Meta-Moment we ask ourselves, *How would my best self respond?*, we will at the very least know how we'd like to behave at this critical juncture. And maybe we'll get close this time and even closer the next.

If we try hard enough, we can begin to embody the emotional attributes most parents say they wish to possess, for the sake of their loved ones and themselves. I often ask audiences to complete the following sentence:

I promise to work toward being a parent who is . . .

Here are the most common answers:

- Passionate
- Encouraging
- Inspiring
- Compassionate
- Patient
- Engaged
- Supportive
- Kind
- Understanding
- Loving
- Responsible

It's a pretty good start. What other words would you add to the list?

Here's another way of approaching the ideal of your best self. In the world—at your workplace, in your community, wherever you are known—you have a reputation. If you're like most people, you take it seriously and do your best to maintain it.

We each have a reputation at home too. The "community" there may be quite a bit smaller than how we usually mean that word. But it still fits the definition. In this community, you have a reputation for being kind or patient or understanding or forgiving, or the opposite of those qualities, or somewhere in between. You're known for being quick or slow to anger, easy or hard to talk to, honest and sincere or snarky and sarcastic. You're famous for keeping your promises or forgetting them, for being generous or selfish. You earned your reputation at home the same way you did everywhere else—by your actions.

So, what's your reputation at home? And what did you do (or fail to do) to deserve it?

Remember, your children have been studying you closely since they were newborns. They've read every vocal inflection, facial microexpression, every gesture and touch and body language clue. They sense the vibe that says more than your words ever could.

Thinking about our reputation makes us behave in ways that cause people to admire and respect us. We're willing to be a little bit better than we might otherwise, all for the sake of reputation. Doesn't your family deserve the same effort you give to the rest of the world? You might think about your response to this question: How do you want your children to talk about you when they're older and looking back?

Another way to effectively regulate our emotions is to remind ourselves in advance when they're likely to require regulation. For many of us, reentering home at the end of the day is a potential flash point. At work, we're on our best behavior, which often means sublimating our natural emotional responses and pretending to be the person who is always calm, competent, and in control. It's hard keeping such a tight leash on our emotions. When that day is done, we experience an automatic release. It's palpable, like a big exhale. We can finally be ourselves.

So here you are, headed home at last. Drained. Harried. Possibly hungry. You reach for the doorknob, turn it, and enter into . . . peace and serenity. Calm and tranquility. The loving, nourishing embrace of your family. A release from all your cares and woes.

Well, maybe that's how it goes at your house. If it does, may I congratulate you on being such a shining exception to the rule.

If that's not your typical experience, you may need to find some kind of reminder—something to warn you, maybe just before you walk in the door, that you need to remain cool for the sake of your family, no matter how severely you may be tested. That doorknob, then, becomes an important part of your emotional life. It's the object that reminds you it's time to regulate your emotions, no matter what you encounter on the other side of that door.

Anything can be your personal reminder. I have a friend whose evening commute takes her past the Golden Gate Bridge. She's made that her signpost—every day when she sees it, she knows it's time to begin lowering her emotional temperature. Another acquaintance lives in Manhattan and uses the Statue of Liberty as his talisman. When he sees it on the way home, he automatically starts to power down and prepare for the place where he'll need all his best qualities.

But all these strategies will work only after we've taken that Meta-Moment. It has to become almost second nature. How long will it take for that to happen? More than a day or two? More than a week or a month? If you try hard and apply yourself and hit the pause button as you formulate your response to whatever just triggered you, maybe in six months it will begin to feel like a habit. It's unrealistic to think the Meta-Moment is going to become automatic overnight. I spend most of my life researching and teaching and discussing emotion skills and the Meta-Moment as a tool of the emotionally intelligent person. Yet after a long day of work, when I get home tired and hungry and brain-dead, even *my* skills sometimes go out the window.

There's another tool we can try that usually succeeds in groups where emotion skills are valued: a *charter*. This is a written document or pact that details how everybody in your home wishes to feel. It also includes a list of commitments that everyone in the family will make to one another to create the best possible home environment. Depending on the age of the children, they may need help with the writing part. But even young kids know the right words to use.

The charter is created by asking three questions. The first is: *How do we want to feel as a family?* This question can be asked over an evening meal or, perhaps, over the weekend when there is some downtime. Some of the words we've seen come up frequently among families are loving, respectful, included, safe, happy, calm, grateful, and playful.

The second question is: *What can we do to experience these feelings as often as possible?* You can get highly specific with responses to this question, such as deciding how you'll set the proper mood when it's time to do homework, or at bedtime, or when dinner is served. Some families make a commitment to saying "I love you" each night before bed.

The third question, which gets answered after the charter has been "lived" for a while, is: *What can we do when we are not living the charter?* Again, it's helpful to get specific. For example, if one family member says something that makes another member feel disrespected, what's the best way to express the feeling and settle whatever dispute might have caused it? Many charters include statements like "We will listen carefully without judgment to the person who feels like the charter has been broken."

Simply allowing everyone to help create a charter is empowering. It gives everyone in the home a sense of agency over their emotional environment. In most households, that alone would be a big step forward.

A charter can benefit parents by accommodating their needs too. After a certain hour, adults want to enjoy peace and quiet and no conflicts or excess noise—so the charter requires everyone to respect those wishes. It's a way of reminding children that their parents are human, too, with the same emotional needs as anyone else. In the long run, that's an important lesson for kids to learn, but too many parents try to shield them from that reality. As an unintended result, children have a hard time acknowledging adults' feelings, let alone respecting them.

Putting our emotional needs in writing has a way of making them real for ourselves and everyone else. It acts as a reminder for those times when we feel overwhelmed. It serves like a contract—a formal agreement drafted in a moment of calm consideration, to help you during moments when you are anything but calm and considerate. You may feel a little self-conscious posting a charter on your refrigerator door or hanging it on a wall. But if you try it, you might find that it works.

I'm reminded of an interview I did with a dad at a RULER workshop. "I reamed my six-year-old son, David," he said. "He walked into the kitchen and started bugging me for batteries for his gaming console while I was in the middle of another bickering match with my wife. I was already pissed and David's 'Dad-Dad-Dad-Dad-Dad-Dad' just sent me over the edge. I exploded and sent him to his room. In fact, I half chased him out of the kitchen and up the stairs."

Next morning, while the kids were getting ready for school, the man saw a note next to David's bed, but the handwriting belonged to his son Jason, who was ten. "It was puzzling," the dad said, "so I picked it up and read it. It was a script, showing David how to manage his feelings. *Take three deep breaths. Daddy was just in a really bad mood. He will feel better tomorrow after he rests.*

"It was a wake-up call like nothing I'd ever had in my life," the man said. "My older son, Jason, was learning in school how to handle emotions, and my wife and I realized we'd not only been terrible role models, but we'd been subjecting both our kids to a lot of unnecessary hurt. When I asked Jason how he thought we should have handled it, he said, 'You know, Dad, at school we have a charter to tell us how we all want to feel. Maybe we should have one for home too.'"

Sometimes, during sessions with parents, I'll drag up a difficult moment from my own childhood—when I failed the test for my yellow belt in Hapkido and I took it out on my parents. We turn this into role-play.

Imagine I'm your adolescent son, and I arrive home after failing my martial arts test. I walk into the kitchen yelling and screaming, "I *hate* you. . . . I *hate* Hapkido. . . . I never should have tried taking that test, you knew I wasn't ready but you made me do it. . . . I'm never going back. And I'm not going to school tomorrow *either!*"

Also imagine I'm likely not getting you at a very patient and under-standing moment. You worked all day, then had your hour-long com-mute home. You're beat, you have the beginning of a headache, you're hungry, and now this. You know I need your help to get through this moment. You want to be the parent who is there for your kids when they feel down and defeated.

But instead my bad behavior triggers yours. You ignore what I'm saying, zero in on how I'm saying it, and start yelling right back. It's a reflex action—like a counterpunch. Here are some of the role-play responses parents offer up:

"You are not allowed to talk to me that way!"

"You need to calm down and lower your voice and stop crying over nothing!"

"You're not going to be a quitter. I paid for those lessons and you're going to take them."

"Don't tell me you're not going to school tomorrow, because you *are*! You'll do as you're told!"

Some parents go to the other extreme to sound conciliatory but still trying their hardest not to engage with this child's disappointment and shame.

"You'll be okay, honey. Those teachers don't know what they're doing."

"You know Mom loves you always, no matter what."

"Look, calm down now and I'll take you to the mall after dinner, we'll get you something fun."

"You don't have to go back if you really don't want to."

And here are some of my favorite responses:

"We'll go buy you a yellow belt this weekend. We don't need to wait for your sensei to give it to you."

"How about if we find you a sexy Hapkido coach?"

"Let's go shopping for some new clothes."

After we stop laughing, we go through what highly skilled parents might say:

"It's understandable. I get it and it stinks. How about we take a walk and talk about it?"

"Just stop a second and take a deep breath. I know how upset you are."

"Let me give you a hug."

"It seems like you need some space to calm down. Do you want to go up to your room for a few minutes and we can talk during dinner?"

After the role-play is over, I ask parents about how they felt when that hypothetical child unloaded on them. Here's what they say:

"Like a bomb just went off."

"Like I need my own time-out."

"Desperate and scared."

"I ask myself, '*Why* did I want to be a parent?'"

And this becomes the *a-ha* moment of the exercise: adults come to the seminar to learn strategies for helping their kids regulate their emotions—and then realize that for that to happen, parents first have to regulate their own.

We can boil the entire process of bringing emotional intelligence into your family down to these four steps.

- Step 1: *Set yourself up for success.* Build your family charter! Consider the words on the charter each day. Those adjectives should always be somewhere in your mind. Remember, you have to take the Meta-Moment and be your best self before you can help a child to regulate. You are the role model. Your facial expressions, vocal tones, and body language matter.
- Step 2: *Explore.* Be the emotion scientist—the learner, not the knower—and listen to understand, not to build your own argument. Remember that behavior is the symptom, it's not the emotion. Validate, show unconditional love and support, help to deactivate if necessary. Don't attribute emotions to your child. Allow them to express their feelings. Listen for themes and help them to label.
- Step 3: *Strategize.* Once you know what your child is feeling and have a sense of the situation, you can support with a short-term

strategy: self-talk, reappraisal, a hug, and just being present. The strategy you might want your child to use might not be the strategy that works best for you. And strategies often bomb at first, so your child needs your support to build this muscle. And have long-term strategies ready—from helping your child to problem-solve to seeking professional counseling.

- Step 4: *Follow up*. Emotion regulation is a lifelong journey. History often repeats itself. Kids need regular check-ins and continuous support. Consider: What are the conditions we can create for our children to support their healthy emotional development? How might my best self support my child? And have compassion for yourself and your child. It doesn't mean letting yourself or your child off the hook. It means you approach setbacks in a more constructive way, learning from them instead of beating yourself up.

Here's a good example of that process from my own life. I have a niece, Esme, who was adopted from Guatemala as a baby by my cousin Ellyn, who has red hair and fair skin. I consider Esme my niece because Ellyn is more like my sister than a cousin. When Esme was in kindergarten in upstate New York, one of her classmates said to her, "Eww, you're a different color than your mother!"

Esme was devastated.

Ellyn called me and said, "She was teased about her skin color. Now she's crying and upset that she looks different from me and the rest of her family and all the kids in her school. She doesn't want to go back to school, she says. She's scared. I knew this was going to happen at some point, but I didn't think it would be in kindergarten. I'm losing it and about to get into my jeep and drive over to this kid's house."

Okay, so the first needed step here had nothing to do with Esme— her mother, Ellyn, had to take a Meta-Moment so she could model a healthy response for her daughter. Because that's how it works—our kids watch us intensely and examine everything we do for clues about how they should behave in similar situations.

Ellyn was triggered, understandably. She was like a mother tiger protecting her cub. But if she freaked out, Esme would get the message that even her mom couldn't handle the situation calmly. If Esme was ever going to find a way to navigate this incident or others like it, Ellyn had to show the way.

I wasn't surprised at what had happened. Research shows that about one-third of American kids are bullied at some point, and appearance is the top reason. Children can be cruel when it comes to looking different.

Still, it hurt to know that my five-year-old niece was being attacked for the color of her skin. Given my own childhood struggles with bullying and the anxiety and fear that followed, I had to help her and her mother.

We all owe it to one another to stop bullying when we encounter it. It's not just a matter of a child being mistreated—peer victimization actually changes the biology of the brain. It disrupts the development of the stress regulation system and related neurocircuitry, leading to a host of problems, from physical and mental illness to difficulties with social relationships and academic challenges. And these effects persist well into adulthood, contributing to problems with employment, relationships, and overall quality of life. Bullying isn't just something that happens in playgrounds or on school buses. Its effects never completely go away.

Meanwhile, most of us will face moments like Esme's at some point during our lives. According to someone, we're too fat or too skinny, our nose is too big, we're too dark, not smart enough, not tough enough. These comments devastate us and stick with us long afterward. The lingering self-hate and self-doubt are lacerating.

When a child hears sentiments like that over and over, soon the voice is coming not from the outside but from inside. She's internalized that negative view of herself. When she feels shame, fear, self-loathing, she'll need help to regulate those emotions—a caring adult to help prevent any negative views of herself from holding her back in life.

If Esme had been able to react like an adult, she would have instantly realized she might have been dealing with a racist family, and she might have said something like "Yeah, my mother and I are different colors, so what? Plenty of families have members who are different colors. But why do you care?"

Instead, those vicious words found their mark. We did our best to support Esme's regulation of her hurt feelings. Ellyn's response wasn't textbook perfect. There was no charter in place to guide her. But she did everything else right. She asked Esme the right questions and listened to her answers, like a good emotion scientist. She helped her daughter strategize future responses she could use if anyone tried to shame her again. She reminded Esme that her family was diverse. We all coached her on go-to phrases she could say to herself when she felt uncomfortable. We reached out to her teacher and school principal. Our goal was to lay the groundwork that would support Esme for years to come. Our immediate intervention was not a quick fix, but the beginning of a journey.

Esme carried that wound for a long time, and it wasn't the last time she was made to feel inferior because she was different. But given the careful attention her mom gave to supporting her healthy emotional development, Esme's now a highly resilient and academically successful high school student.

Often, when we're under psychological assault, our default position is surrender—we accept that this negative view of us must be true, and we adopt it as our own. Children do not have the inner strength or knowledge about people and their motivations to be able to say, "Who are you to define me? What gives you the right? Why do you need to belittle me? I reject you and your judgment of me—I know who I am." They need our unconditional adult support.

· · ·

As I've said before, the permission to feel begins with the question that Uncle Marvin had the courage to ask me: "How are you feeling?" Likewise, its denial begins with the failure to ask it.

When our children don't have the permission to feel—they still will. But those feelings will go on in the dark, and the pathways between those feelings and their visible manifestations and behaviors will become almost totally obscure. Not only will our children suffer—we'll also have no idea why. (I doubt that scenario sounds unfamiliar.) However, when we support our children to be their full, feeling selves, we'll see how deeply and enduringly they can flourish. And it starts with us as their role models.

10

Emotions at School:
From Preschool to College

During seminars for educators I'll usually ask, "How many of your students receive a comprehensive emotion education from pre-K through high school?"

They all look at me as if I'm from another planet.

Then I'll ask, "How much did *you* learn about emotions in your own schooling?"

I get back a similar look, one that says, You *really* have to ask?

And when I ask what they learned during teacher training about the role of emotions and emotion skills in education, here's what they say:

"I learned how to teach my subject."

"I learned how to make a lesson plan."

"We discussed how to establish an orderly classroom."

"We read a chapter on bullying prevention."

Later, when I speak with those teachers one-on-one and ask how they infuse emotions into the classroom, here's the typical answer:

"Honestly, I make it up as I go."

Unfortunately, that approach is not working very well. If it were, all of our schools would be thriving havens of positivity filled with emotionally healthy teachers and students. Many are not.

The teaching profession is known for being highly rewarding *and* extremely taxing. The pressures of high-stakes testing, large class sizes, supporting a diverse range of learners in their classrooms who have complex needs, inadequate wages, and administrators who are not always supportive contribute to high attrition rates—40 percent of teachers leave the profession within five years, and in some communities the rate is as high as 30 percent annually.

In a survey we distributed to more than five thousand teachers, we found that 70 percent of the emotions they reported feeling each day were negative—mainly "frustrated," "overwhelmed," and "stressed." This is especially troubling because teachers who experience more negative emotions are also more likely to have sleep problems, anxiety, and depression, be overweight and burned out, and have greater intentions to leave the profession.

Those negative emotions also have serious ramifications for students: teachers who are stressed offer less information and praise, are less accepting of student ideas, and interact less frequently with students. If we want children to flourish, we have to begin taking care of our teachers.

As mentioned previously, when we asked twenty-two thousand high school students across the United States, "How do you feel each day in school?," 77 percent of their responses were negative. The three most frequent answers were "tired," "stressed," and "bored." Among all students, LGBTQ students reported the greatest anxiety and depression and the least positive feelings such as acceptance and psychological safety. LGBTQ youths in the United States experience greater rates of bullying, lower academic achievement, and higher dropout rates than their non-LGBTQ peers.

Many of the high school students we surveyed reported feeling that their schools gave little thought to creating an atmosphere where students can actively participate in their education, where they're expected and encouraged to think about a lesson and find meaning in it. One study in Connecticut discovered that thirty-nine thousand students were either disengaged or entirely disconnected from school. It's no wonder that by high school so many students are tuned out.

And as much attention as bullying gets, it continues to go on unabated. Students who are bullied report feeling fear and hopelessness while in school. You'd hope that schools would know how to deal with these extremes of emotional distress, since they happen under the eyes of teachers and administrators. But on the contrary, most teachers report feeling unprepared to deal with classroom bullying. Teachers also miss most incidents of bullying because of where and how it occurs, are unlikely to interfere in disputes between students, and when not trained in emotion skills often base their disciplinary strategies on what they themselves experienced in their childhood at home. The result: A lot of children go unprotected from bullying, as I did. They go through the school day feeling so afraid and ashamed that they can't fully focus in class or develop academically or socially. Even the bullies are ill-served—they tend to have emotional or psychological problems of their own, which go unaddressed and unmediated without appropriate teacher training. And schools are known to overreact to challenging behavior by confusing normal conflicts with bullying or relying on harsh interventions, especially with preschool children and African American boys.

One in five American children is experiencing a mental health issue such as depression or anxiety, and over half of all seventeen-year-olds report having either experienced trauma directly, ranging from neglect to abuse, or witnessed it at least once as a child. By failing to recognize trauma's effects on learning, educators risk compounding the trauma and jeopardizing students' prospects in school. For many children, school might be the only place any of these issues are recognized and addressed.

So even before the doors open, we know there are challenges to creating an atmosphere where all children will feel ready for learning.

It's true—we can't change every child's home environment. But research shows that the presence of a caring adult allows a child to manage stress more effectively. Yet in a study of two thousand teachers, only about 50 percent said they have strong individual relationships with their students. In the same study, two thousand students also were surveyed and only 34 percent reported having such relationships.

Traditionally, feelings and behavior mattered to teachers primarily when students failed to sit still, be quiet, pay attention, and remember what they were taught. Although misbehavior was addressed—disciplined and punished, for the most part—the underlying causes, which are nearly always emotional, were left untouched.

Consider the fact that classroom corporal punishment is still allowed in nineteen states, and suspensions and expulsions, disproportionately applied to black students, have continued to rise. Problems are exacerbated when instructors and staff misunderstand students' emotions and behavior or are unaware of their own biases. And when teachers are not given the support they need and are asking for, there's little reason to hope for improvement.

"From a Nation at Risk to a Nation at Hope" is the title of a January 2019 report from the Aspen Institute's National Commission on Social, Emotional, & Academic Development. It's worth quoting here. It reads:

> The promotion of social, emotional, and academic learning is not a shifting educational fad; it is the substance of education itself. It is not a distraction from the 'real work' of math and English instruction; it is how instruction can succeed. It brings together a traditionally conservative emphasis on local control and on the character of all students, and a historically progressive emphasis on the creative and challenging art of teaching and the social and emotional needs of all students, especially those who have experienced the greatest challenges.

All true. Yet when I talk with administrators, principals, and teachers about the role of schools in providing students with a social and emotional education, here's what I hear:

"We don't have the time or training to deal with the social and emotional challenges my students are facing. They're too complex."

"I don't want our school to spend time teaching about emotions, because that will take away from AP classes and affect whether our students qualify to get into the top universities."

"I'm here to teach. Leave these issues to parents, the ones who *should* be dealing with emotions."

Their fears of what might happen if there's an emotional aspect to education are unfounded. In fact, students are grateful to learn that their teachers are human beings with feelings too.

David Brooks, the *New York Times* columnist, wrote that once, when he was teaching a college course, he announced to his class that he had to cancel office hours to deal with some unspecified "personal issues." Ten or fifteen students emailed him to say he was in their thoughts and prayers. For the rest of the term, he wrote:

"The tenor of that seminar was different. We were closer. That one tiny whiff of vulnerability meant that I wasn't aloof Professor Brooks, I was just another schmo trying to get through life. That unplanned moment illustrated for me the connection between emotional relationships and learning."

He continued:

"A key job of a school is to give students new things to love—an exciting field of study, new friends. It reminded us that what teachers really teach is themselves—their contagious passion for their subjects and students. It reminded us that children learn from people they love, and that love in this context means willing the good of another, and offering active care for the whole person."

Emotion as a part of the learning experience doesn't simply mean that students and teachers will bare their souls and grapple with difficult emotional issues. It also means that students will engage more fully with what they're learning.

Related to this, in two studies we conducted with fifth and sixth graders, we found that when the classroom climate was rated as warm and supportive by outside observers, children reported feeling more connected to their teacher, there were fewer conduct problems, and students' grades were higher.

A colleague, Mary Helen Immordino-Yang, neuroscientist at the University of Southern California, reminded me of a self-evident principle we often forget: Children learn what they care about. They're no different from adults in that regard. We can try to force them to absorb a lesson, but we're not going to accomplish much. Some kids may be able to commit facts to memory and regurgitate them on demand, but that's not the same thing as learning.

Earlier I discussed how brain scientists have found that depending on our emotional state, our chemical and hormonal profiles change dramatically and our brains function differently. The three most important aspects of learning—attention, focus, and memory—are all controlled by our emotions, not by cognition. Immordino-Yang's research shows that when students feel deeply engaged and connected in the learning process, and when what they learn is relevant and meaningful to their own lives, there is activation in the same brain systems (for instance, the medulla) that keep us alive.

Students have no problem addressing emotion skills in the classroom. In fact, they love it. I recently watched a room of fifth graders practice putting RULER skills to use. I told them about the day when I was around their age and failed my karate test and how shattered and dejected I felt. Then I asked them to come up with some emotion regulation strategies they might have suggested had they been my friends that day.

"I would tell you jokes," one student said.

"Okay, that's interesting," I said. "It might lift my mood, at least. What else?"

"I would say let's go get ice cream," said another.

"That would definitely improve my mood," I said, "but what would happen if we did that every time I was disappointed or sad?"

"We'd get sick or fat!"

"Very possible," I said. "What else could you do?"

"I would say keep trying . . . because you miss one hundred percent of the shots you don't take," said another student, quoting the hockey legend Wayne Gretzky.

"I've never heard that line, but I really like it," I said. "That might help me feel better, but what if I'm feeling more hopeless than sad? Like I never will pass the test."

"I'd want to know which moves you messed up," said another student, "and I'd help you practice them."

I wasn't looking for a right answer—I just wanted them to run through all the possible emotion regulation strategies they could imagine.

Meanwhile, their teachers were witnessing this in disbelief. Later, they told me how insecure they were about their ability to teach emotion skills until they realized how much those skills resemble science, math, or any other academic subject. The goal isn't to tell children what to feel or what specific strategy to use to regulate—it's to turn them into caring citizens who are emotion scientists, with tools for gathering important information and putting what they discover to good use.

At the end of the class I said to the students, "Thank you for letting me into your classroom. Does anyone have questions or final thoughts?"

One student said, "I really liked the lesson because *I* was involved."

A boy named Kevin raised his hand, which his teacher told me he never does.

"What would you like to share?" I asked him.

"Sir," he said, "I just wanted you to know that you remind me of myself."

The teacher couldn't believe it. I was deeply moved. Later that afternoon, I learned that Kevin lived across the street from school, alone with his alcoholic mother. He didn't like going home, I was told, because most of the time no one else was there. You can just imagine the emotional issues Kevin brings into the classroom. Is there even a chance that his academic performance is not affected?

I've mentioned my uncle Marvin before and made clear, I hope, what a huge influence and inspiration he's been for me. His presence is in everything I do in my work, but especially when it comes to the role of emotions in the classroom.

Uncle Marvin was a middle school teacher in upstate New York for two decades. He had unusual success with the kids who passed through his sixth-grade classroom. Back then, there were no controlled experiments to confirm his observations, but many of the students he kept track of made it through high school and college without becoming derailed, even in the face of major obstacles.

Marvin had figured out instinctively that something was often missing in a child's journey toward success—the ability to embrace and use emotions wisely. He knew that if we grew up acquiring emotion skills, they would make us better learners, decision makers, friends, parents, and partners, better able to maintain our health and well-being, deal with life's ups and downs, and achieve our dreams.

I knew firsthand, from a young age, that his ideas worked, because they made it possible for me to navigate the extreme bullying and loneliness in my early life. Without him, I would never have made it through middle and high school.

Fast-forward ten or so years. I graduated from college with a major in psychology but was teaching martial arts and working in sales, uncertain about my professional path. That's when I came across the landmark book *Emotional Intelligence* by Daniel Goleman, published in 1995. There was a chapter about the burgeoning field of social and emotional learning (SEL), a term used to describe school-based programs to teach emotional intelligence. A light bulb clicked on. SEL was exactly what Uncle Marvin had been teaching in his classroom way back in the 1970s.

I called my uncle immediately, and within a few weeks we had begun to write a curriculum for middle school students. Together, we were going to marry his decades of experience as an educator with the new psychology of emotional intelligence and transform the schoolhouse.

Goleman's book also introduced me to two researchers, Peter Salovey at Yale University and Jack Mayer at the University of New Hampshire. They were the psychologists who had written the seminal 1990 article on emotional intelligence that formulated the concept itself. I contacted each of them, and they agreed to meet me. At lunch with Salovey, I shared my enthusiasm about writing and testing the curriculum Uncle Marvin and I were creating.

"What's your theoretical model?" he asked me. I had no clue what he was talking about. I had been out of college for a couple of years and had no formal background in social science research.

That year, I got rejected from Yale's doctoral program and accepted at the University of New Hampshire's. Marvin and I continued to work on our curriculum throughout my graduate school years and even more once I eventually got to Yale to work with Salovey as a postdoctoral researcher.

There, I met Edward Zigler, a renowned child psychologist who was known as the father of the federal Head Start program. He was one of the few psychologists at Yale who had a background in public school education. I explained what Uncle Marvin and I were trying to do.

"What's your logic model?" he asked me. Again, I was stumped. I had no idea what he was asking. I thought I had learned my lesson from Salovey and read up on all the theories of emotion in graduate school. But now I had my second wake-up call. I needed to show *why* and *how* RULER would lead to better outcomes for kids and adults.

By 2004, our middle school curriculum was finally finished and ready to be tested. My uncle and I were off like the Wright brothers, trying to make a difference in the world. Marvin flew up from his home in Florida, and together we started recruiting schools and training educators. We had some small successes here and there, but for the most part, here's what we heard:

"Teaching kids about anxiety makes me anxious."

"I'll teach words like happiness and excitement, but I'm not opening the Pandora's box to anything else like despair and despondent."

At one school meeting, a principal said, "You're going to turn the boys into homosexuals." An experienced teacher then said, "My job is not to talk to you *or* my students about feelings," and stormed out. "Does anyone have *another* perspective?" I asked the room. After everyone finished laughing, a young male teacher shouted, "Sir, I was actually a student in this school, and she was *my* teacher. I really wish she would have stayed for this."

At another seminar, a teacher came up to me during a break and said, "Nothing you could say today could help. I'm emotionally bankrupt!" I couldn't stop thinking about what his students must experience in class. Will they develop curiosity and passion? Will they be engaged? Will they even learn?

To be clear, Uncle Marvin and I had some successes, but implementation of our curriculum was uneven at best. The message became more and more apparent: educators were mostly uncomfortable talking about emotions—their own *or* those of their students.

And the leaders set the tone of the school or district. They can make or break any program.

A group of teachers took me aside at an early RULER training and said, "We love this, but our principal has already told us we can't start RULER until after the state tests." I remember thinking: It's August, and the state tests aren't until March. We're all wasting our time.

The CEO of one network of schools said to me, "I want my students to learn facts, not feelings. In my schools, there is no place for feelings. Just teach them to sit still during tests." Ironically, while leaving that school, I overheard a kindergarten teacher yelling at a five-year-old, "Zip it! Go to your seat! We're not friends anymore!"

I left there in shock, wondering, How safe can that child feel in this school? How inspired? How much will that child actually learn today?

In the end, Uncle Marvin and I failed. We were too narrow in our approach. We failed because we focused solely on the students. The missing piece was educators' own emotion skills. In hindsight, it makes perfect sense.

Over time, we learned, as with everything for children, it takes a village. If children are to develop emotion skills, *all* the adults around them need these skills too.

Several years ago, I created an award in honor of my uncle, to recognize educators who exhibit outstanding teaching practices on emotional intelligence. One of Uncle Marvin's former students heard about it and sent me a letter to forward to him. Here, with permission, is what she wrote:

Dear Mr. Maurer,

I am sending this note with the hope that you are well and enjoying the important work that you continue to do with your nephew in the realm of empowering students and teachers.

The class I had with you in 6th grade was, to this day, one of the most meaningful educational experiences I have ever had. Your kindness and ability to personalize learning has inspired me throughout my life in countless ways.

I currently teach second grade in NY and am working on a degree in Educational Administration. I am driven by my desire to fix a broken education system. My focus is on the continuous inequities in standardized testing and the lack of acknowledgment of children's social and emotional needs in the classroom. Unfortunately, we have to justify wanting to teach in a way that allows children to discover who they are as people and learners, and show how powerful it can be when a child's feelings and needs are honored and celebrated. (No easy task, as you know.)

I have two beautiful boys, Jonathon, 11, and Henry, 9. They are both sensitive and kind. As Jonathon begins his middle school adventure in September, I reflect fondly on my experience in your classroom, and only hope that my son can make a similar connection to a teacher that will empower him and teach him the way you taught me.

Quite a tribute to Uncle Marvin and what he tried to accomplish. Compare that with the letter I received from the head psychologist of a network of schools—the same network whose CEO said he wanted students to focus on facts, not feelings. Here, with permission, is the letter:

Hi Marc-

I think that the major roadblock to the successful rollout of RULER and our other SEL initiatives is the lack of training and understanding of child development, social-emotional health, and appropriate expectations and needs of students by the people that are making the decisions. Very few people at the top have any training in these areas.

I was told just yesterday by a principal that nobody in our network cares about a child's confidence, emotional well-being, mental health, integrity, overall success as a person (characteristics I brought up specifically)—they only care about test scores. That is what they are judged on, and that is the message that they are sending to our kids. The focus is punitive ("effort" academy during recess and after school for children who don't have high scores or who make errors like not underlining the evidence or finishing in the time limit) with the expectation that teachers should use "a punishment so severe" that the children never engage in those behaviors again. My questions about this approach were met with a comment about whether or not this is the right place for me since that is the direction the network is moving.

That's what we're up against.

. . .

Thankfully, many educators have begun to recognize what's missing. According to a 2018 survey by McGraw-Hill Education, an overwhelming majority of administrators, teachers, and parents believe that SEL is just as important as academic learning. But at the same time, 65 percent of teachers said they need more time than they currently have to teach emotion skills. The most effective educators recognize that social, emotional, and academic learning are intertwined. Yet there is a disconnect between what we expect teachers to know about SEL and the offerings of teacher training programs in colleges and universities. Few teacher preparation programs fully integrate SEL into the curriculum.

So what exactly does a school that prioritizes SEL look like? That's been the big question in educational circles over the past two decades or so, ever since we realized that many kids and schools were struggling with problems such as violence, drugs, inadequate learning, and teacher attrition.

Here's a definition: It's a school where "children and adults understand and manage emotions, set and achieve positive goals, feel and show empathy for others, establish and maintain positive relationships, and make responsible decisions."

That definition comes from a group called the Collaborative for Academic, Social, and Emotional Learning (CASEL), which was formed in 1994 with the goal of "establishing high-quality, evidence-based social and emotional learning as an essential part of preschool through high school education." SEL recognizes that three intertwined factors—cognition, behavior, and emotion—must all be considered in order to create emotionally healthy environments where learning can take place. According to CASEL, when that happens, children are able to "build self- and social-awareness skills, learn to manage their own emotions and behavior (and those of others), make responsible decisions, and build positive relationships."

Since the inception of CASEL, numerous approaches and programs have emerged with the goal of creating an equitable education system for all children irrespective of race, ethnicity, gender, sexual orientation, language disability, family background, family income, citizenship, or tribal status. Not all have succeeded. Some attempted only to teach children self-esteem, thinking that would be enough. It turns out that giving kids unmerited praise backfires and can even decrease intrinsic motivation. Other programs have focused on teaching scripts like "I feel . . ." statements, where teachers and children are told to declare their emotions using sentences beginning with those two words. But these statements alone don't guarantee everyone will develop emotion skills or that SEL will be embraced as a consistent part of teaching and learning.

The best SEL approaches are systemic, not piecemeal

SEL has to have buy-in from the top and the bottom. If the principal is less than completely committed, teachers will get the message, and students will be shortchanged by half-hearted efforts. Leaders need to make room for ongoing professional development—all the adults in the school must learn the skills so they can be role models for kids. Teachers at each grade level need to understand social, emotional, and cognitive development and be steeped in culturally responsive pedagogy. Teachers have to recognize that they're the students' primary role models during the school day. Not just when the subject is SEL—all the time. And students must have a voice in how SEL is implemented; if it's not relevant and meaningful to their particular circumstances, it will fail.

Research shows that teachers with more developed emotion skills report less burnout and greater job satisfaction; they also experience more positive emotions while teaching and receive more support from the principals with whom they work. The presence of emotionally intelligent leaders also makes a difference. When school leaders have emotion skills, the teachers in their buildings report feeling more inspired, less frustrated and burned out, and more satisfied with their job. In turn, teachers' relationships with their students are warmer; their class-rooms are better organized and managed and more supportive; and they use more practices that cultivate creativity, choice, and autonomy. And when children have better relationships with their teachers, they are more engaged and committed to school, adjust better socially, and are willing to take on more challenges and persist in the face of dif-ficulty. They also disrupt less, focus more, and perform better academi-cally.

SEL can't be addressed only in a ten-minute morning meeting or every Thursday, fourth period. It can't be isolated in occasional assem-blies for students or in workshops for teachers. SEL has to be an ev-eryday thing—it has to become part of the school's DNA. There needs to be a common language among all stakeholders. SEL has to be in-tegrated into leadership, instruction, faculty meetings, family engage-ment, hiring procedures, and policies.

In regard to classroom instruction, students watch their teachers closely, paying attention to each facial expression, every gesture, the rise and fall of their voices. They're constantly picking up information on how teachers feel about the topic, about teaching, about them as students. That emotional subtext exists in every lesson ever taught—whether the teacher intends it or not.

If students are going to learn, they need to feel the teacher's emo-tional investment. History can be boring or it can be exhilarating. Geometry can be confusing or awe-inspiring. Foreign languages can shut students down or open doors to exciting new worlds. The subjects themselves don't change, the emotion the teacher infuses into the les-son does.

At the best RULER schools, every adult walks the walk—not just teachers, principals, and guidance counselors but also security per-sonnel, cafeteria workers, janitors, and bus drivers. There's a school in Seattle where the attendance officer has a huge Mood Meter on the wall behind her desk. The kids often race into school late and flustered. When they enter her office, she slows them down, and they plot their feelings. That alone has a way of calming students' nerves. Together they explore different strategies to help them prepare emotionally to enter the classroom. In some schools, there are even Mood Meters on the buses, and as kids board, they check in and consider whether that's a helpful emotional space for beginning the school day.

Even the building has to be part of the effort. I'm thinking of the schools I've visited where, right inside the entrance, the vision and mission statements make it clear that SEL is part of the education, and there is a huge Mood Meter with feeling words in multiple languages. Inside classrooms, there are student creations reflecting a strong commitment to the diverse backgrounds of students, including self-portraits surrounded by adjectives representing their best-self attributes.

Classroom seating arrangements also have an influence. How creative or inspired would you feel if you spent all day sitting and staring at the back of a colleague's head? Typical school architecture sends an emotionally rigid message of its own. Schools need to allow for some flexibility and acknowledge the human need for connection with our peers.

Beyond the classroom, we've collaborated with organizations such as Playworks, which helps schools to figure out how to integrate SEL into recess with games and sports. And we've worked with the Boys & Girls Clubs of America to expand opportunities for SEL skill building to after-school time. I often think about how scared and unsafe I felt on the playground during recess and in my after-school program and what would have been different if the adults in these spaces were emotion scientists.

Comprehensiveness also means SEL goes home. When I was a kid, conversations with my parents about school went something like this:

"How was school?"

"Fine."

End of discussion.

But in schools that engage families, conversations go more like this one, which was shared with me by a parent:

"Hey, Mom, I just learned a new word, *alienation*, because we are studying the civil rights movement. We had to think about what makes us feel alienated. I thought about the time I wasn't chosen to be on the baseball team. It was the worst feeling to be left out and not know why. What makes you feel alienated, Mom?"

"Actually, honey, it's a really good question. I feel that way a lot of the time at work. I'm the only female officer in my precinct, and so I don't get invited to do a lot of things with the other officers."

That mother told me that she hadn't really thought about how isolated she felt at work until her son started her talking. Not only did it help them bond, but it was a big moment for her personally. As a result, she decided to talk to her lieutenant about it.

The best SEL efforts are proactive, not reactive

Being proactive means we don't wait for problems to arise and then deal with them—we adopt measures to prevent them.

Not many kindergartners will raise their hands and say, "Excuse me, I don't feel emotionally supported in this classroom." Most high schoolers won't go to the principal to complain, "I feel anxious and fearful during most of my classes, and I need some strategies to deal with that." Our schools have to take the initiative. They have to make it clear to every student that emotion skills are an integral part of their education.

How does that work? In practical terms, at some point during the first couple weeks of school, a teacher might say, "Everyone, we all know that emotions matter, so let's talk about the feelings that we all want to experience as students in this classroom." That opens up the discussion for building their *Emotional Intelligence Charter*. The point of the exercise is to have students describe how they want to feel, including how they'll help one another feel those emotions, to give them control over their classroom environment. In some schools this means a shift in mindset, from following rules to creating an emotionally safe space of their own. It's an act of hope, a switch from a passive to an active voice.

Younger children say they wish they felt happier, safer, calmer. Older students have more nuanced needs: they want to feel empowered, respected, motivated, supported, trusted.

In every grade, students love it—being asked for their input is something of a novelty. All day long, year after year, their emotions are bottled up, and suddenly here comes a teacher wondering what they're feeling, how they want to feel, and what they'll do to get there.

Leaders, teachers, and staff go through the same process. Typically, they'll say they wish to feel more valued, appreciated, inspired, connected, and supported. Many of their desired emotions are the same ones named by students. It makes me wonder: Is there something missing in the school environment as it's been constructed over the course of decades and centuries—something both students *and* teachers need?

The information that is gathered is then turned into a visual display—often a large, creative poster—which everyone signs. Once that's complete, and routines are formed, adults and kids are more willing to share feelings and speak up when they feel the need.

Here's an example. "We were playing at recess and another girl—she was new—came over and tried to join in," said Callie, an eight-year-old from Seattle. "We didn't really want her to play with us, but then we thought about our classroom charter and how all of us agreed that everyone should feel *included*. If we didn't let her play with us, then we'd be breaking the charter, and she would feel bad. If the same thing happened to us, we would feel left out and lonely. So, we made room for her to join. We had a lot more in common with her than we thought."

The most effective approaches integrate SEL into the curriculum and provide skill building across *all* grade levels to reach *all* children

Of course, how SEL is taught and learned depends on age, but there is no age at which it is too early or too late to start. And when students come to school having lived through multiple traumatic events or from homeless shelters or temporary housing, as one in ten New York City public school students do, they often require additional support from a school psychologist, social worker, or counselor.

SEL needs to be culturally responsive. For example, in New York City there are more than 160 different languages spoken by students and their families. Programs that are developed within a Western culture may not address cultural subgroups adequately and might even alienate students from different backgrounds, because how people express and regulate emotions varies greatly across cultures.

The most comprehensive SEL interventions focus on developing social and emotional skills through classroom topics, conversations, and activities that relate to students' interests, needs, relationships, and lives—in and out of school. For example, in one RULER classroom I visited in Tulsa, a book about the Holocaust, *The Boy in the Striped Pajamas,* was used to teach emotion skills. Students tracked and analyzed different characters' emotions throughout the story, providing evidence from the text for the possible causes and consequences of the emotions and their impact on each character's decision making and relationships. Students also made connections to their own lives and their larger community.

Development matters too. The way our brains process emotions and emotion skills is inextricably linked to our social and cognitive development. For example, five-year-olds might learn about sadness and pride, fifth graders about hopelessness and elation, and middle schoolers about jealousy and envy.

In secondary school, SEL needs to match the unique developmental needs of adolescents, who want more autonomy as they explore topics such as identity, relationships, and decision making. At a Los Angeles middle school, students created a Mood Meter journal to track their feelings at the end of each class for two weeks and then analyzed the data, including the causes and consequences of their feelings. The goal was to look for patterns of emotions related to time of day, day of week, and subject area in school. Students also monitored their sleep, exercise, and eating habits to help them make greater inferences from their own data. Then they considered helpful emotion regulation strategies and made other recommendations for how they could perform at their best. The project culminated in a personal plan to enhance student well-being. It also was a great example for how SEL can be integrated seamlessly with English-language arts, math, science, or health classes—and the real world.

At the heart of our high school approach is helping students answer three big questions. The first is: Who am I? Here, students explore their personality traits and motivation, among other competencies. The second question is: What do I want out of my high school career? Here, students explore their goals for their relationships, academics, and extracurricular activities. The third question is: What do I need to achieve my goals and support my well-being?

Students continue to learn strategies to build empathy and for managing interpersonal conflict. Jorge and Ali were close friends at a Chicago high school. As with other fifteen-year-old males, their joking often became physical. On the way to soccer practice, Ali was texting a new girlfriend. Jorge tried to see, but Ali wanted his privacy. He raised the phone high over his head, shouting, "Dude, cut it out! You're worse than my little brother."

Jorge forced Ali's arm down, grabbed the phone, and dashed through the locker room door, taunting Ali to catch him. Ali's backpack got caught on the door handle, and while he struggled to free himself, Jorge decided to rub it in by throwing a dirty sneaker at him.

Immediately, Ali tore himself out of his backpack, leaving it swinging from the doorknob. He ran toward Jorge in a rage that stunned everyone in the locker room. The coaches had to pull Ali off Jorge as he was about to punch him in the face.

The boys were brought to the administration office.

"Guys, I know you're good friends," the assistant principal said upon entering the office, "and you know we have tools for dealing with this. Ali, you sit here outside of the office, and Jorge, take that empty chair in the waiting area. Let's take some calming breaths and then I'm going to ask you to complete these 'Emotionally Intelligent Blueprints,' and I'll come back for you in about five minutes."

The lists of prompts on the blueprint required each boy to say how the other might have felt, the possible cause of the feelings, and how each of them expressed and regulated their emotions. The act of taking each other's perspectives helped Jorge and Ali move from the red quadrant to the green, so they could begin to think clearly.

When they were finished, the assistant principal brought them back together and said, "Okay, let's hear what each of you wrote. And remember, no interruptions or judgment."

Ali explained that in Iraq, where he was born, throwing a shoe at someone was the worst possible insult you could hurl. As he spoke, Jorge realized his mistake. "I'm really sorry. I truly didn't know. I won't do it again. I promise," he said.

Ali and Jorge collaborated on strategies they could use in the future to manage their feelings more effectively. As a follow-up, the boys worked together on a class presentation comparing Middle Eastern and Spanish cultures, making it a restorative practice for them and the class.

In addition to classroom content, we've collaborated with Facebook to build inspirED, a free resource center to elevate student voices and empower high school students in creating positive changes in their schools and communities. Students follow a four-step process, with resources and tools to support each phase: (1) Assessing their school climate with a variety of measures; (2) Brainstorming passion projects to serve their school communities; (3) Committing to and completing a plan; and (4) Debriefing their successes and impact.

The best SEL approaches pay attention to outcomes

Monitoring the progress and impact of SEL is an integral part of implementation. Is it working? Are people delivering the lessons? Are expected outcomes improving?

Over the last decade, evidence has accumulated for RULER's positive impact on students' emotional intelligence skills, social problem-solving ability, work habits, and grades; on classroom and school climate, including fewer instances of bullying; and on teacher stress, burnout, and instructional support for students. Two meta-analyses have also demonstrated that a systematic process integrating SEL is the common element among schools that report improved relationships between teachers and students, a decrease in emotional challenges and problematic behavior, and an increase in academic success. The benefit can even be measured in dollars and cents. In 2015, a benefit-cost analysis of six SEL interventions in American schools found that the ratio was about eleven to one. A benefit-cost analysis compares the monetary cost of an investment (implementing an SEL program) with the monetary value of its outcomes (for example, education attainment). This means that, on average, for every dollar invested in SEL, there is a return of eleven dollars, a substantial economic return.

The difference between schools that embed SEL and those that don't can be endlessly studied. But there's one example that never ceases to move me.

A boy named Jordan had transferred into a RULER school from an elementary school where he was horrifically bullied. As part of a RULER lesson, he was assigned to write a poem about the word *isolated*, using it in the context of his feelings—almost like a letter to the bullies who once tormented him. He wrote the poem but was afraid to share it—he feared he'd be bullied all over again. His teacher, who was trained in RULER, asked him if she could share the poem with her colleagues. Reluctantly, he agreed and got compliments, which gave him the courage to read his poem aloud to his fellow students.

Here, with his permission, is his poem:

You're ugly
I know
I have been told this

You're silly
I know
I have realized this
You look like an alien
I know this has been pointed out to me
You have big eyes
I know I have looked in the mirror
You can't be a pilot
You're not smart enough
It is possible. I have considered this
With every insult you invent it's strange but it's true
You point out my many failings
And help me to improve
As you highlight my many weaknesses you also highlight my strengths
My openness leads to my kind personality
My silliness brings laughter to the world
My resemblance to movie aliens only highlights my intelligence
My big eyes portray my feelings and widen my view
I may not make it as a pilot, but I could be
You see, every insult you invent gives me a view into your mind
And although I have many problems, I feel sorry for you
Why oh, why do I feel sorry for you?
Because your mind cannot break free
The wall of insults you build limits your mind and feelings
So soon if you don't stop, you'll turn inhuman
And have the biggest problem of all
Loneliness
Think about it

Within seconds of Jordan reciting the last line, his classmates shot straight out of their seats, teary eyed and clapping—a standing ovation he never expected.

"We can't believe this happened to you," one told him. "It's not like that here." Once he realized that his new school was a safe haven, Jordan blossomed.

In fact, when I visited the school a year later, I ran into him in the cafeteria. He told me excitedly, "I'm doing a lot of writing, and I think I want to be a poet." When I nodded, he came back with a large stack of papers and a broad grin. Before he turned away, he said confidently, "Look for me on the bookshelves."

Had Jordan been in a school that wasn't devoted to SEL, perhaps he would have found a sensitive teacher who would recognize what he needed after his previous horrible experience. But, perhaps not—in which case he'd likely go the rest of his life without ever confronting what had happened to him or knowing that he could and should feel safe and a worthy contributor to society. If we truly believe in the mission of SEL, Jordan's poem is a testament that key outcomes go far beyond test scores and must include how students feel in school.

And how do all the issues we see in schools play out once our kids get to college? Pretty much how you'd expect.

According to a report by the Center for Collegiate Mental Health, between 2009 and 2015, the number of students who visited campus counseling centers increased by more than 30 percent. Anxiety and depression are the top reasons students seek out counseling.

In 2018, the World Health Organization released findings from a study of nearly fourteen thousand students from nineteen colleges in eight countries. More than one in three students reported symptoms consistent with at least one mental health disorder, mostly depression, anxiety, and substance abuse. The 2018 Healthy Minds Study found that 23 percent of college students are taking psychiatric medication, up from 18 percent in 2016. In another survey, 87 percent of college students said they "felt overwhelmed," and 63 percent said they "felt very lonely."

In my own nonclinical research, especially at Ivy League institutions,

I've found that at the beginning of a semester, college students experience a healthy mix of pleasant and unpleasant emotions—excitement and anxiety, happiness and exhaustion, pride and fear. But by midterms, they mostly feel stressed, overwhelmed, and frustrated. When I probe for the reasons, they say things like "I don't believe you can be successful without being stressed," or "I must persevere at all costs," or "I have to look out for number one." Their strategies for managing these emotions—sleep deprivation, excessive video-gaming, poor eating habits, drug and alcohol consumption—are not helping. Recently, I asked students to share how they hoped to feel at college. The top answer was "loved." When I asked why, they said, "I feel manufactured," "I feel like an impostor," "I don't know who I am." I was floored.

Our traditional approach has been to address students' mental health issues after the fact. They are diagnosed with anxiety or depression or say they are thinking about suicide. Then they are offered medication or therapy. But colleges, like primary and secondary schools, need to take a preventive approach. How will there ever be enough resources to provide counseling for all of the college students who need it?

But integrating SEL into higher education is a challenge. Unlike the K–12 setting, where it's easier to take a systemic approach, the college or trade school structure presents bigger obstacles for teaching SEL skills, given the sheer size of student populations and the distant nature of relationships between faculty, college counselors, and students.

As a result of how higher education is structured, piecemeal approaches abound: some colleges have created "relaxation stations" that include massage chairs and beanbags, while others offer yoga and mindfulness classes. But a more systemic approach is absent.

I've found that students often arrive at college with interesting mindsets about SEL training. For example, I've taught a university course called Emotional Intelligence for nearly a decade. It's classified as an academic course, but my goal is to teach students evidence-based practices to support their well-being and to help them develop the "soft" skills employers are asking for. But I get serious pushback from many students. In my class here is what I've heard:

"I didn't need these skills to get into Yale."

"Now you want me to put emotion regulation on my already long to-do list?"

"I took this class to learn about the science of emotional intelligence, not to practice breathing exercises!"

At that point I needed a Meta-Moment to stop myself from saying, "You might not have needed them to get in, but you'll need them to get out." Instead, I explained how only 42 percent of top employers believe new graduates are adequately prepared for the workforce, especially with respect to social and emotional sills. One survey, "The Class of 2030 and Life-Ready Learning"—conducted in collaboration with Microsoft and McKinsey & Company's Education Practice—suggests that 30 to 40 percent of today's jobs will require social and emotional competencies. I also explain that among college students there is a "restriction of range" of IQ scores, which means that IQ no longer has much predictive value. In other words, it's not a high IQ that gets you places. It's the social and emotional skills that give today's college students the competitive edge.

If university students are to achieve the benefits of SEL, they must be convinced that learning and practicing the skills makes a difference. At Yale, my colleague Emma Seppälä, author of *The Happiness Track*, and I have piloted a few SEL interventions. In our first study with more than two hundred undergraduates, students reported less stress and burnout, higher self-compassion and acceptance of their emotions, and greater school engagement after a six-week intervention. In a pilot study conducted by a graduate student in public health, sixty-seven students were divided into two groups. One group (the intervention group) was asked to track their moods, using our Mood Meter app, up to six times per day, for four weeks. The other group (the control group) did "business as usual" (until after the study, when they got the same access to the Mood Meter app). The intervention group also attended a weekly two-hour class focused on developing emotional intelligence skills, practicing self-care, and goal setting. Compared with the students in the control group, those in the intervention group had significant reductions in depression, stress, and anxiety and a significant increase in self-rated mindfulness (for instance, feeling more present). This year, we are launching our first ever randomized controlled trial to test the effectiveness of our approach.

What's most telling from the study were student anecdotes:

"I learned that being vulnerable opens up wonderful opportunities for friendships and deeper connections. I learned that sometimes you have to be as gentle with yourself as you are with others, and be as understanding with others as we are sometimes of ourselves."

"I wish this class could continue as long as possible because I fear that this peace that I feel will drift away, but I must have hope that I will take the lessons with me always."

"Calm, serenity, focus, and overall happiness are all within my reach, so long as I interiorize the wisdom gathered in this workshop."

"This class gave me a sense of waking up from a long dream. I had this feeling of not actually being alive or 'here' for many years, and now I feel that I am out of my slumber. If I had to describe the way I saw my life in colors, before it would be a pale gray, and now it would be a bright white. Almost as if I had a new blank canvas to put vibrant colors on, this workshop taught me that one can improve and detoxify oneself through putting attention and awareness on one of the most basic principles of living."

What I hear in all this is a cautionary tale: We're not doing these kids justice in supporting their emotional development. So by the time they're young adults in college, they're suffering from the absence of an education in emotions.

Whether it's cyberbullying or guns, pressure to do drugs or to be thin, helicopter parents or neglectful ones, learning differences or identity struggles, our kids' brains are overwhelmed with emotion, cutting off pathways to higher reason and learning . . . unless they know how to handle all of the emotions that come along with these situations. And when kids are on a hamster wheel of achievement—test scores, volunteering, tutoring, advanced placement classes—it puts SEL at the bottom of the list.

SEL is the universal life jacket, keeping students afloat and open to learning. Only when children learn in psychologically safe environments that nurture their emotion skills can they can move from helplessness to resilience, from anxiety to action, from scattered to centered, from isolated to connected.

But, as my colleague Dena Simmons, assistant director of our center, has espoused, SEL must be grounded in a larger context of equity and justice efforts to ensure *all* children, especially the most marginalized, have the opportunity to thrive and take greater control over the direction of their lives. With SEL, we can raise youths who are academically strong as well as kind, compassionate, resilient, and successful, all at the same time. We can raise kids who are able to collaborate, follow through, and bounce back after failing. With SEL, we can model and teach that confidence, vulnerability, passion, and achievement are inextricably linked.

Over the years, our center has moved from working with individual schools and districts to building citywide and statewide approaches. In New York City, we have trained and coached nearly every superintendent. At present RULER has been integrated into about a quarter of the seventeen hundred public schools. In Connecticut, with generous support from the Dalio Foundation, Hartford Foundation for Public Giving, Seedlings Foundation, and Tauck Family Foundation, among others, and in collaboration with policy makers and organizations such as the Connecticut Association of Public School Superintendents and Connecticut Association of Boards of Education, we have launched an initiative, "Making Connecticut the First Emotionally Intelligent [Education] State!" Our goal is to bring the principles and practices of SEL into every school and after-school program in the state, to ensure that all five hundred thousand–plus students, eighty-five thousand educators and staff, and families benefit from an education in emotion skills.

Until SEL permeates the entire school village and community leaders become a vocal, energized force for SEL, it won't occupy its proper place. This is the tough lesson Uncle Marvin and I learned: only when everyone demonstrates that SEL matters will politicians, school boards, and administrators pay attention and make the necessary effort. That commitment filters into the classroom, the cafeteria, the gymnasium, the playground, the school bus, to the principals and teachers and aides and guidance counselors, to parents, and, ultimately, to the benefit of all.

When we unlock the wisdom of emotions, we can raise heathy kids who will both achieve their dreams and make the world a better place.

11

Emotions at Work

IT'S EASY TO SEE why the workplace might be an emotionally challenging environment.

After all, we spend half our waking hours there, surrounded by people we didn't choose to hang around with and who don't necessarily share our habits, our values, or our tastes. And yet we need to get along with them, and find a way to cooperate and collaborate, or risk being unhappy—and possibly unsuccessful—adults. The very means by which we support ourselves and our families is dependent on how we perform in this arena. And unlike at school, in the workplace there's no graduating—we're in this for the long haul, as in decades. We'll enter in our youth and exit, most of us, on the cusp of old age.

No wonder the emotional stakes are so high.

We think of work as being driven by skill sets and information, by brainpower and experience, and by the hunger for achievement and accomplishment. All those things are in the mix, of course. But emotions are *the* most powerful force inside the workplace—as they are in every human endeavor. They influence everything from leadership effectiveness to building and maintaining complex relationships, from innovation to customer relations. In chapter 2 we discussed how our cognitive abilities—what we focus on, where we devote our efforts, what we remember, how we make decisions, our levels of creativity and engagement—all depend on our emotional state. And as we've seen in chapters 4 through 8, our ability to use those emotions wisely—to recognize, understand, label, express, and regulate them effectively— often determines the quality of our relationships, health, and performance.

So let's start by thinking about the moment you wake up. Are you glad at the thought of getting out of bed and off to your job, or do you want to pull the covers over your head and hide? Picture the handful of co-workers with whom you come into contact most often. Do you smile at the thought of these encounters or groan inside? In the office or shop or factory, do the hours fly by as you immerse yourself in the challenges and pleasures of your job, or are you watching the clock and praying for a fire drill? Those are all unmistakable signs of your emotional state while at work, which will have a major impact on how you feel and behave even when you're not working.

Now ask yourself: How accurate are you at identifying your own and others' emotions while at work? What feelings do you experience most often each day? Are you aware of what causes you—and your colleagues—to be in the yellow, red, blue, and green? What are the unwritten rules in your workplace to guide how emotions are expressed? Which expressions are acceptable? Frowned upon? How much emotional labor is required to meet your work demands? How skilled are you at regulating your own emotions and supporting others in regulating theirs?

A woman I know was in the habit of arriving early at the office and starting work while the place was silent and empty. She loved the solitude and accomplished a lot in a short amount of time, but once her colleagues punched in, it was a different story. When she was forced to interact with her co-workers, she got more and more drained, and the hours began to drag. Often, after work, her husband would suggest dinner out, but most nights all she wanted to do was go home and de-compress alone, with a book and a glass of wine.

After going through our training, she realized what was happening: she would start work in the yellow quadrant, energized and positive, but gradually move into the green and then, by the end of the day, into the blue—low energy and negative. That emotional shift was taking its toll on her marriage and her home life. It was time to begin regulating her feelings throughout the day, to employ the strategies necessary to avoid ending each day in the blue. That way she would have enough cognitive resources to devote to her job *and* maintain a healthy rela-tionship with her husband.

That just underscores how much our work lives and our emotional lives intersect and commingle. It doesn't matter if you're the CEO of General Motors or you work at a car wash, your emotional needs—to belong and feel seen and heard—are the same. And just because you're twenty-five and brilliant and just got hired at Goldman Sachs or Face-book doesn't mean you excel at emotional intelligence or will be able to function optimally at home *or* in the workplace.

Today especially, when so many jobs require the ability to commu-nicate, our emotion skills determine how we'll perform. If we can't rec-ognize and understand our own feelings, label them, and then express and regulate them successfully, we'll struggle. Many of us are inter-acting with other people—colleagues, customers, counterparts at other firms—and if we can't empathize with them, and use that information to co-regulate *their* emotions, we won't be effective. If we can't find grounds for friendly collaboration, it will be almost impossible for most of us to do our jobs well.

On the surface, all our workplace interactions are about work—we're in a planning meeting, we're exchanging information about a new project, we're sharing research on a joint venture, negotiating a con-tract, exploring a partnership. But those interactions take place within relationships often forged in nonwork moments: a bit of small talk on the elevator, or swapping restaurant advice, or sharing some office gossip, and so on. A workplace is a community like any other. The professional friendships born of personal moments make our work easier and more pleasant or the opposite.

Your new colleague is a joy to be around and has made your job more enjoyable than you thought possible? Wonderful. Your boss is a manipulative bully who likes making your day difficult? Not so good. These are typical workplace minidramas, and like it or not, you're involved—emotionally. You'll have to take the bad with the good and deal with it. Developing emotional intelligence will help. And creating an emotionally intelligent ecosystem will yield even greater benefits.

Everything that happens at work is, at heart, an emotional moment. "I deserve a promotion" means I think I'm worth more to you than you realize (and if I don't get that new title, I'll feel unappreciated and look for another job). The tenor of our face-to-face encounters, the location of my office, how you greet me on the elevator—these all are expressions of how you feel about me, which will determine how I feel about you.

"Businesslike" is a total misnomer—beneath the veneer of our corporate mission, business is anything *but* businesslike.

Research shows that our emotions and moods transfer from one person to another and from one person to an entire team—both consciously and unconsciously. It's called "emotional contagion," and its study dates back to the 1890s. Someone smiles and you smile back, or someone frowns and your expression changes, and suddenly you feel happy or sad without knowing why. Sigal Barsade, a professor at the Wharton School, University of Pennsylvania, conducted the first study to test whether emotion contagion occurred in groups and whether it subsequently predicted people's behavior in the group. Study participants were randomly assigned to four different groups, each representing one quadrant in the Mood Meter. A trained confederate, acting as a participant, was assigned to each group to elicit the appropriate feeling. Participants were told they were playing a manager who was responsible for negotiating a bonus for an employee. Each group also knew they had a fixed pot of money and needed to consider what was best for both the employee and the company. Results showed not only that the confederate elicited the emotional contagion but that it also influenced subsequent behavior. Specifically, participants in the yellow and green quadrants reported less conflict, greater cooperation, and better individual performance, and they even allocated money more evenly compared with the participants in the red and blue quadrants.

As we develop emotion skills, hopefully we become more aware of how we are actively creating emotional contagion and understand its impact on others. We also need to ask ourselves: Am I generating the best emotion to achieve the best outcomes for our group?

Recently I interviewed my colleague David Caruso on the role of emotions in effective leadership. It's critical, he said, to match the emotion to the task at hand. He talked about a product development meeting he attended where the manager was energetic and positive. His mood was infectious and useful during the brainstorming part of the meeting. But later, when the group turned its attention to detailed product plans and market data, that same enthusiasm wasn't so helpful. The high-energy, confident vibe that encouraged creative new ideas re-sulted in a launch schedule that was overly optimistic and riddled with hasty mistakes. This was a case of an emotion not facilitating the kind of problem solving required. After realizing what had gone wrong, the team leader changed the emotional tone of the room but did it in a way that was barely detectable: she used the tone of her voice and the cadence of her speech to lower the energy level and provided examples of the importance of getting details right. This allowed the product manager to slow his thinking, become more reflective, and check his assumptions. Emotions, Caruso said, flow throughout organizations. Leaders must understand the role of those emotions in influencing how people decide, think, and work toward their goals.

The organization itself must also enable individuals to influence emotions. "Having the skills is one thing," Jochen Menges, a leadership scholar at the Universities of Cambridge and Zurich, shared with me recently. "But it's another to be able to apply the skills at work." According to his research, emotionally intelligent workplaces are distinguished by how people *behave* at work, and that behavior is heavily influenced by *structure*—the way people are organized, meaning hierarchies—and by *culture*—what people believe is appropriate. If the people in charge are not drawing on their emotional intelligence in how they convey themselves and manage others, who will?

But if emotional intelligence is so necessary in the workplace, how are we supposed to acquire it? In school, emotion skills can be integrated into the subjects already being taught. After all, education is school's sole purpose. It's trickier to develop new emotion skills in the workplace. When exactly would that training happen? During our coffee breaks? Over lunch? A yearly retreat? We're not at work to learn—we're there to *do*. Businesses have invested millions into "emotional intelligence training and development programs." But I've yet to see a *comprehensive* program in an organization that helps employees improve their emotional intelligence in a way that builds lasting habits. That's one reason I cofounded Oji Life Lab, which offers emotional intelligence training to businesses. In a carefully designed sequence of bite-size learning steps, learners develop emotion skills through a wide range of thought-provoking activities including fast-paced videos, an interactive Mood Meter, personal reflections, and engaging exercises. The program even includes live video discussions with a trained coach, in both group and one-on-one settings. By exploring emotion skills over time, people retain more and develop habits that become automatic.

Even when modern organizational thinking attempts to introduce these skills into the workplace, employers often resent it for taking time and focus away from the bottom line. Many managers still don't get it—that the bottom line depends on a workforce that's motivated, energized, and committed to a common goal.

I recently spent some time consulting at a company where the relationship between two key executives was causing a serious problem.
Both were skilled and good at their jobs. But one was by nature anxious, and she took every reaction and feedback to heart. The other was
a loud, outspoken man who always said whatever came to mind, without stopping to think how it would be received. You can see how that
combination might clash, and it did. Neither of them had the emotion
skills to recognize what was going on and attempt to control the situation by talking it out and regulating their reactions to each other. Every
interaction was tense and not as productive as it should have been.

That left it to their supervisor to try to mediate these very different
temperaments. Not exactly how the boss wanted to spend her time, but
if she didn't help those two regulate their emotions, the work in their
department would have suffered.

These interactions play out constantly in business situations. Think
about what happens when you sense that a co-worker is in a foul mood.
It immediately changes the office vibe. No one wants to get too close.
Communication falters. There's a nervous pall over everything that
saps the psychic energy from the place.

Or there's a supervisor who dampens all enthusiasm and crushes
all creativity. In meetings, he greets every dissenting opinion with a
piercing glare and a grimace. His subordinates figure, why bother trying? Soon, they go from discouraged to disengaged. They're spending
time on Facebook instead of developing new ideas. Before long, they're
online looking for new jobs.

Business schools devote semester-long case studies to significant
business flameouts. But do they ask whether a lack of emotional intelligence and related skills had anything to do with them? It's important
for them to do so, given all of the research on the impact of poor emotion skills on how employees feel and operate. To be sure, some business
schools, including the Yale School of Management and the University
of Zurich's Graduate School of Business, have begun investing in developing students' emotional intelligence. But none are accustomed

to factoring emotional intelligence into their thinking about students' success and failure, and no wonder—there are no numbers to rely on, no charts or graphs to provide reliable answers (yet).

When you look into the research on the inner life of workers, the results are cause for worry.

With support from the Faas Foundation, which funds efforts to create healthy, safe, and fair workplaces, a team at our center, led by senior research scientist Zorana Ivcevic Pringle, has conducted numerous studies on the role of emotions in the workplace. In one study we surveyed one thousand people and in another fifteen thousand people. Both studies had a demographically representative sample from across the United States.

Among the many questions in the studies, we asked these two: How are you feeling at work? What are your experiences like at work? Participants provided their answers to these questions *in their own words* in addition to completing surveys.

Here's what we found:

- About 50 percent of workers used the words *stressed, frustrated,* or *overwhelmed* to describe their feelings at work.
- About a third of workers indicated that they felt happy or proud less than 50 percent of the time they are at work.
- Many of the things they shared that caused them to feel unpleasant emotions were related to other people—colleagues not taking their jobs seriously, administrators lacking good decision-making skills, co-workers slacking off, and people lacking empathy/listening skills.

We also asked subjects for three words to describe what they would most like to feel at work. "Happy" was the number one choice. That came as no surprise—in all my work with various groups, whenever

I ask how people would like to feel, the first word out of everyone's mouth is "happy." It's like the default choice, the one that we blurt without much thought.

But it was the number two and three choices that were most revealing. After *happy*, respondents said they wanted to feel *excited, joyful, appreciated, supported, fulfilled, respected, inspired, accomplished*. The word *valued* was another top choice, and women were about twice as likely as men to use it. That list indicates what's most lacking in the typical workplace.

Other research supports our findings:

- According to a 2018 Gallup survey based on a random sample of 30,628 full- and part-time U.S. employees, over half are "not engaged" at work—while another 13 percent say they have miserable work experiences. The estimated cost to businesses is $450 billion a year in lost productivity.
- In the nonprofit sector, 45 percent of young employees insist that their next job will *not* be in the nonprofit sector, citing burnout as one of the main reasons.
- Thirty-five percent of employees surveyed say they routinely miss three to five workdays a month owing to job stress.
- Forty-five percent of physicians say they feel burned out. Recently, I asked a large group of medical residents to consider a typical day and how they felt throughout it. Then I asked them to summarize the experience in one word. Seventy percent of the residents shared terms such as *meh, bored, polarized, overwhelmed, stressed,* and *pensive*. Only 30 percent used words such as *content* or *calm*.
- According to a Stanford University study, more than 120,000 deaths annually may be attributable to workplace stress, which accounts for up to $190 billion in health care costs. The stressors include a lack of health insurance, work-family conflicts, and inequitable treatment.

Recent research shows that when it comes to burnout and engagement, it's not either/or—it can be both. Julia Moeller, formerly a researcher in our center who is now an assistant professor at the University of Leipzig, led a study that focused on the burnout rate of the best, most capable workers. Those employees suffer burnout precisely because of their high levels of engagement; they are so committed to their jobs, and so good at them, that they wind up with more responsibilities than they can handle—and rather than turn down assignments, they continue to accept them until they are completely overwhelmed. In a related *Harvard Business Review* article by Moeller and Emma Seppälä, who leads our center's college student well-being work, they described a woman whose task it was to organize an ambitious conference for her company, and she did a great job, except that

> in the last weeks prior to the event . . . her stress levels attained such high levels that she suffered from severe burnout symptoms, which included feeling physically and emotionally exhausted, depressed, and suffering sleep problems. She was instructed to take time off work. She never attended the conference and needed a long recovery before she reached her earlier performance and well-being levels. Her burnout symptoms had resulted from the long-term stress and the depletion of her resources over time.

Meanwhile, as that Gallup poll found, half of all workers feel just the opposite—unengaged. Clearly, there's a precise emotional balance that must be struck—employees must be sufficiently engaged to do a good job, but not to such an excess that it causes burnout.

Part of avoiding burnout is encouraging workers to speak up when feeling pressured or unfairly burdened. But that doesn't happen in isolation—the freedom to express yourself, positive or negative, has to be a part of the everyday experience. When I teach in Yale's Executive Education program, I'll often ask: "Are you comfortable expressing your authentic emotions at work?"

"No!" most reply without hesitation.

"I think it is dependent on whom you are speaking with or whom you are negotiating with in a meeting," said one audience member.

"I might say something to a team member or a colleague that I would most certainly *not* say to the CEO," said another. "Like, I would never say, 'Jeremy, you really embarrassed me in that meeting, let me tell you why.'"

They were both saying the same thing: that at work they'd rarely, if ever, express how they felt to the people who could do something about it.

Owing to my role as the director of a center, I know firsthand the impact of suppressing emotions in the workplace.

Do you know the one thing that keeps me up at night? How my employees feel. That should haunt the sleep of every CEO, supervisor, manager, and boss in the world. It's the prime determinant of virtually everything that will happen in an organization—good and bad. If we're an emotionally intelligent workplace, most challenges (though not all) are manageable; if we're not, everything is a struggle.

Before we hire someone at the center, I know that they have the experience, talents, and brains necessary to do the job. But I have little to no idea whether they possess emotion skills. Will they know how to get along with their new co-workers and collaborate, without rivalries or competitiveness getting in the way? Can they adapt to a new environment and contribute but not disrupt? Will they be able to empathize with clients and understand how to interact in a way that serves their needs as well as those of the organization? If not, we're doomed to fail. If the people make the place, as Benjamin Schneider of the University of Maryland once wrote in a famous essay, then surely an organization would be much better off if the employees had emotion skills.

As a company grows, it becomes even more vulnerable to the lack of emotion skills. Here's an example. Years ago, I hired someone as a supervisor, and this person decided it would help if he shielded me from any work-related complaints that his team might have had. Perhaps he thought he was doing me a favor. Maybe to some misguided executives this might have seemed like a good thing. But it was a disaster. For a variety of reasons, my colleagues had become progressively more dissatisfied in their jobs, but no one was letting me know. Things went on that way for a while until this supervisor left, at which point employees felt free to come forward and express to me the feelings they had been forbidden to share. We had become an emotionally dysfunctional workplace, and it showed in the work itself. It took over a year for the place to return to normal. If an institution that bills itself as a center for emotional intelligence can be afflicted by poor emotion skills, it can happen anywhere.

The lesson for me was that I needed to make myself more vulnerable by expressing my own feelings more often and to more of my colleagues. Only if I did that first would they feel safe expressing themselves to me. I had to learn to operate with less authority and more humanity.

Another example from my own workplace: Years ago, I had an employee who consistently looked uninterested and apathetic. She was difficult to read, but she got the job done. So I did my best to accept that and regulate my emotions when I was around her. Then we had a meeting with a school superintendent, and this employee sat there looking conspicuously bored. I was seething the entire time. It was so bad that after the meeting ended, the superintendent said to me, "What's up with that woman?" I had to assure him that we were interested in working with him. It shows how one person's emotional state and lack of skills—even a subordinate's—can infect an entire workplace.

It took me weeks to figure out how to speak about it with that employee. I didn't have the language or an opening to discuss with the employee how she seemed to the rest of us. But once I did, I learned that she was suffering with depression and in need of help. In that situation, it was tempting to be an emotion judge—*What's wrong with this woman, is she rude or something?*—instead of an emotion scientist who genuinely wanted to know what was going on. Back then, we still hadn't come up with a charter for the center, one similar to the family and school ones described in the previous chapters. Today, when there is a disagreement or something feels off, the charter acts as our guide for how to identify and address even uncomfortable feelings.

As Jack Welch, General Electric's legendary management guru, said, "No doubt emotional intelligence is more rare than book smarts, but my experience says it is actually more important in the making of a leader. You just can't ignore it."

Emotional intelligence has attracted considerable attention among organizational behavior scholars. Stéphane Côté, a professor at the Rotman School of Management, University of Toronto, has summarized a couple of decades of research that demonstrates that emotional intelligence, measured as a set of skills, correlates with a wide range of important workplace outcomes, including the following:

- Creativity and innovation
- Organizational commitment
- Job satisfaction
- Customer service ratings
- Managerial performance
- Social support from team members
- Leadership emergence—the extent to which someone not in an official leadership position exerts influence over colleagues
- Transformational leadership, including greater motivation and inspiration
- Job performance, particularly in jobs requiring more emotional labor
- Merit pay

It's important to note that emotionally intelligent managers and leaders need not always be "nice" bosses. Often they need to use emotion skills to perform difficult, delicate tasks. Emotional intelligence in the workplace doesn't merely mean providing comfort and sympathy; sometimes it requires the ability to deliver difficult feedback to help people build greater self-awareness and skills. We may even need the ability to have challenging conversations about sensitive subjects that will cause hurt feelings. That requires emotion skills too. Emotion skills help us to foster successful workplaces and to correct them when things go awry, as they inevitably will.

Recently, our team developed a measure to assess supervisors' emotionally intelligent behavior to examine whether supervisor skills were predictive of employees' feelings and behavior at work. Survey questions included "My supervisor understands how their decisions and behaviors affect how others feel at work" and "My supervisor is good at helping others feel better when they are disappointed or upset." Prior research has found that employees tend to agree in their reports of supervisor behavior.

Here's what we found: Inspiration, respect, and happiness are about 50 percent higher, and frustration, anger, and stress are 30 to 40 percent lower when there is a supervisor with strong emotion skills. We also found that employee engagement, feelings of purpose and meaning in work, and creativity and innovation are significantly higher and that burnout, unethical behavior, and fear of speaking up when there's a problem or when we think there's a better way to do something are all significantly lower when there is a manager with strong emotion skills. Another noteworthy finding: Employees who are afraid to speak up or feel forced to do something unethical are significantly more likely to miss work and have greater intentions of leaving their job, not to mention the toll it takes on their mental health.

Turnover is the one thing most intelligent businesspeople truly dread. It's a huge drain on any organization. Having consulted with many firms, I can guarantee that if there's higher than normal turnover, it's usually because somewhere there's a bad boss. As the saying goes, "People don't leave jobs, they leave bad bosses." While many business leaders would say that a bad boss is one who doesn't deliver results and a good boss is one who exceeds expectations, I would add that a bad boss is one who is low in emotional intelligence, while a good boss is high in it. We all use the term *corporate culture* as shorthand for the DNA of a company. A big part of that is its emotional state, which begins with the emotional intelligence of the people in charge. And for leaders with high emotional intelligence to be successful, they also need to be placed in organizations with a workplace culture that allows these leaders to use their emotional intelligence.

If you're one of those bosses who thinks emotional issues are nonsense and have no place in the office or at the plant or in the store, I can practically guarantee that you're having trouble keeping good employees. If you can't deal in a healthy way with your own emotions, you probably won't be able to deal with anyone else's.

Having said all that, I must add that there are plenty of successful businesspeople with spectacularly bad emotion skills. Not to speak ill of the dead, but Steve Jobs was a notoriously difficult person to deal with, and it's hard to knock him as an executive. Corporate America is replete with bullies and megalomaniacs occupying the corner offices. They are successful if the only measure of success is making money.

So perhaps you *can* bully your way to the top of a thriving business, but you're going to be lonely up there. And if you look around and think your employees are functioning well, you're blind to the fact that they could be operating at an even higher level had you bothered to pay attention to the emotional state of your workplace. Imagine what Steve Jobs could have inspired in his employees had he possessed some emotional intelligence. Perhaps Apple wouldn't be suffering from the lack of innovation and creativity it has experienced in the years since his death.

When I do seminars for business leaders, I show them the data and I say, "Look here, employees say they feel inspired about twenty-five percent of the time when they have supervisors with low emotional intelligence and seventy-five percent of the time under managers with high emotional intelligence. So what does this tell us?" That's a huge difference. Think of productivity and all the creative ideas that will exist in the emotionally intelligent workplace, and now ask yourself why they don't exist in those other companies.

As I've worked in the corporate world, what I've learned is that creating change in these environments is a daunting task—no different from the obstacles Uncle Marvin and I faced when trying to bring change to schools. The kids were always open to it. The adults, not so much. At work, it's the employees who are most likely to embrace the idea of better emotion skills, while their supervisors are skeptical.

There have been times when I was hired to run seminars at workplaces and heard comments like this, from the big boss who did all the hiring: "Oh, no, *I'm* not going through the training. I want you to teach the people who report to me how to deal with their emotions to become better workers. I don't think I need to change anything—I've already proven I'm successful." Another time a hedge fund executive said to me, "Do you really think we're going to sit around a table and share our feelings?" (Later, talking to someone else at his firm, I heard that he once told her, "It doesn't matter how *you* feel—your job is to represent *me*.")

Research shows that high-power individuals tend to be less responsive to the emotions of people around them. In one study, these individuals responded with lower compassion than people with less power when listening to someone describe suffering.

I talked recently with a woman who's running a major nonprofit. She's brilliant. The chairman of the board is a famous guy. She hates her job for one reason—the way he makes her feel. "He's such a big personality that I'm always second-guessing myself," she said. "I always wonder if maybe he's right and I'm wrong about things, just because he expresses his opinions with such force, where I always have my doubts. He says things like 'Why are you so sensitive?' I go home every night depressed and anxious. I've been an executive and I've run big companies for over a decade, but this is driving me crazy, to the point where I might have to quit."

Over the years I've heard from many people in business who feel this way. They're hired to do a job, but they're being undermined and hampered by a superior who thinks that's a good way to maintain control. Of course, it's not—it simply damages the entire organization.

Had this woman taken a Meta-Moment to calm her anxiety and collect her thoughts, she might have realized that this guy was intentionally messing with her and then devised a strategy for dealing with that. She could have sat him down and expressed her feelings, which may or may not have been productive. At the very least she would know soon enough whether there was any hope for improvement.

If she wasn't willing to do that, my advice was to enlist support from the rest of the board and find a way to get the chairman to back off. And if the board wouldn't support her, she needed to find a better job, because this situation was never going to change.

Fortunately for everyone involved, she finally found strategies to help her regulate her feelings of anger and anxiety and had the difficult conversation with the chairman, expressing what she felt and why. She also went to the board and said that structural changes would have to be made if they wanted her to stay. The chairman relented and has changed the way he treats her, and the board took her suggestions, so she is still there—a much happier, and more effective, executive.

In a 2014 research article titled "What's Love Got to Do with It?," the authors, Sigal Barsade from the Wharton School, University of Pennsylvania, and Olivia O'Neill from George Mason University, showed data supporting that particular emotion's power to transform the workplace. They put forth the idea that "feelings of affection, compassion, caring, and tenderness for others" are beneficial even among work colleagues, creating what they call "a culture of companionate love."

At companies where that type of culture is weak, they write,

expressions of affection, caring, compassion, or tenderness among employees are minimal or non-existent, showing both low intensity and low crystallization. Employees in cultures low in companionate love show indifference or even callousness toward each other, do not offer or expect the emotions that companionate love comprises when things are going well, and do not allow room to deal with distress in the workplace when things are not going well.

Once, in the context of corporate cultures, notions like that would have seemed absurdly touchy-feely. Today, however, respected companies such as Southwest Airlines, Pepsi, Whole Foods, Zappos, and a long list of others espouse those values and even enumerate *love* and *caring*—using those words—in their stated management principles. A study led by Andrew Knight, a professor at Washington University in St. Louis, which surveyed more than twenty-four thousand employees from 161 firms, showed that businesses in which positive emotions prevail have significantly lower levels of employee exhaustion and fewer sick days. Another study found that amplifying positive emotions at work reduced employee burnout and absenteeism and increased commitment, but suppressing negative emotions did just the opposite and decreased customer satisfaction.

Other research shows similar results—that customer outcomes such as the intention to return to and recommend a store to a friend are greater when employees display more positive emotions. But it has to be genuine. If employees are faking the good feelings without actually feeling them, the impact on the customer is lost.

The evidence is clear: businesses that wish to remain relevant and competitive in the workplace can't ignore the power of emotions. In our work at Oji Life Lab, we hear from many people about the benefits of the emotion skills explored throughout this book. Professionals who were once anxious at work now use regulation strategies to find relief. One doctor shared that before he had learned the RULER skills it hadn't occurred to him that he had agency over shifting his emotional states. He shared, "Mindful breathing and reappraisal have drastically shifted my ability to be present and work collaboratively with my colleagues, especially when there is tension in the operating room."

According to Susan David, author of *Emotional Agility*, business leaders throughout the world are starting to realize that by attending to emotions, they can improve both their employees' well-being *and* their organizations' success. And the students now developing emotional intelligence in schools will soon join the workforce and select their future employers in part based on how it will feel to work for them.

In the workplace, we often face a trade-off—it's either a job doing something we enjoy, in an environment that feels supportive and creative, or it's one where the emotional satisfactions are few (or nonexistent) but the money is too good to turn down. There are entire professions that count on the willingness of intelligent, educated people to endure high levels of stress and exhaustion in exchange for the big payday. At some point, most of them discover, no matter how much they were paid, it wasn't worth the toll it took.

So when we're being considered for a job, among our main concerns—beyond the usual inquiries about salary, working conditions, room to advance—we should wonder about the emotional atmosphere where we'll be spending so much time and energy. We might even just come right out and ask, "Honestly, how does it make *you* feel to work here?" Beyond possibly startling the interviewer—though maybe in a good way—we're sure to get some interesting, useful replies.

The message for employers and managers in all this is unmistakable. In today's workplace, top employees will gravitate toward firms that acknowledge emotion's power to foster positive, productive environments. They'll quit bad jobs, leaving behind co-workers who may be no less miserable but who are—for whatever reasons—unwilling or unable to find employment elsewhere. That thought alone should encourage companies to take emotion skills seriously.

Creating an Emotion Revolution

At the end of my seminars, I often ask people to imagine a world where all leaders, teachers, and children are taught emotion skills—where colleges and universities, teacher preparation programs, medical and law schools, sports teams, police departments, corporations, and so on are trained to value emotional intelligence. What would be different if everyone was taught to be an emotion scientist? Here's what kids, parents, teachers, and business professionals have said over the years:

- Everyone would listen more and judge less.
- Fewer kids would be living in poverty.
- There would be less stigma and racism.
- Emotional intelligence would be as important to education as math, literacy, and science.
- All emotions would be appreciated, especially the negative ones.
- There would be less self-deception.
- Feelings would be seen as strengths, not weaknesses.
- More people would be their authentic, best selves.

- Schools would be places where students spend time reflecting on their purpose and passion and developing the skills they need to make their dreams come true.
- People would leave their workplace thinking, I can't wait to return tomorrow.
- We'd see less self-destruction and greater self-compassion.
- There would be less bullying, a greater sense of belonging, and more harmonious relationships.
- Depression and anxiety rates would be dramatically reduced.
- Families and schools would work together to support kids' healthy development.

My personal favorite was one third grader's answer. He said, "There would be world peace!" That's the promise of giving children the permission to feel.

With emotion skills, we will create a more inclusive, compassionate, and innovative world. The science is there to show why this is the missing link in well-being and success. Keeping emotion skills separate from our lives at home, in school, and at work harms us all. We need to launch an emotion revolution in which the permission to feel moves us in ways we have yet to imagine.

When the friendship between passion and reason can freely exist, it will mean greater equity as emotion skills level the playing field for all children, regardless of race, class, or gender. For adults in the workplace, it will mean that collaboration functions seamlessly; no one will ever have to use words such as "synergy," "team building," or "creating a leadership pipeline" again, because emotion skills will turn these concepts into reflexes.

Developing emotion skills isn't about attending a workshop, going on a retreat, or adopting a "program." It's a way of life. It's about recognizing that how people feel and what we do with our feelings determines, to a large extent, the quality of our lives.

A commitment to developing emotion skills means providing extra resources to neighborhoods and communities in need, reducing, at last, wide swaths of harm. Communicating through the lens of emotion skills no longer leaves room for toxic masculinity, feminine objectification, and prejudice of all sorts. It means rolling back policies that create widespread inequality, rethinking violence-saturated media, and revising harmful approaches to discipline, punishment, and bullying. And it means policy makers must join families and educators in tending to the "gardens" in which our children grow.

When I share stories about my childhood, people often say, "But you made it somehow, even with all of the pain. If it weren't for your pain, you might not be doing what you are doing today."

It's possible, I reply. Maybe even probable.

"But I was fortunate," I say. And then I ask a few questions.

How many kids will have parents who recognize their inability to help their child and seek therapy for him? How many will have an uncle who happens to be a pioneer in thinking about the importance of emotional intelligence and can provide unconditional love and support? How many will study the martial arts? How many will dedicate their lives to emotion science? My hunch is not many. If we just hope for the best, many children will fall by the wayside.

Emotion skills are the key to unlocking the potential inside each one of us. And in the process of developing these skills, we each, heart by heart, mind by mind, create a culture and society unlike anything we've experienced thus far—and very much like the one we might dare to imagine.

It's not easy to change a whole society. But we have to try.

Our future—and our children's future—depends on it.

References

Prologue

Adkins, A. (2016, January 13). Employee engagement in U.S. stagnant in 2015. Gallup Inc. Retrieved from https://news.gallup.com/poll/188144/employee -engagement-stagnant-2015.aspx

Anti-Defamation League. (2017). ADL Audit: U.S. anti-Semitic incidents surged in 2016–17. Retrieved from www.adl.org/sites/default/files/documents/Anti -Semitic%20Audit%20Print_vf2.pdf

Gallup Inc. & Healthways Inc. (2014). Gallup-Healthways Well-being Index. Re-trieved from https://wellbeingindex.sharecare.com/

Helliwell, J., Layard, R., & Sachs, J. (2019). *World Happiness Report 2019.* New York: Sustainable Development Solutions Network.

Kelland, K. (2018, October 9). Mental health crisis could cost the world $16 tril-lion by 2030. Reuters. Retrieved from www.reuters.com/article/us-health -mental-global/mental-health-crisis-could-cost-the-world-16-trillion-by-2030 -idUSKCN1MJ2QN

Lipson, S. K., Lattie, E. G., & Eisenberg, D. (2018). Increased rates of mental health service utilization by US college students: 10-year population-level trends (2007–2017). *Psychiatric Services, 70*(1), 60–63. doi.org/10.1176/appi.ps.201800332

Substance Abuse and Mental Health Services Administration. (2018). *Key substance use and mental health indicators in the United States: Results from the 2017 National Survey on Drug Use and Health* (HHS Publication No. SMA 18-5068, NSDUH Series H-53). Rockville, MD: Center for Behavioral Health Statistics and

Quality, Substance Abuse and Mental Health Services. Retrieved from www
.samhsa.gov/data/

1. Permission to Feel

American Psychological Association. (2018). *Stress in America: Generation Z*. Stress
in America Survey. Retrieved from www.apa.org/news/press/releases/stress/2018
/stress-gen-z.pdf

Centers for Disease Control and Prevention. (2018, June 7). Suicide rates rising
across the U.S. [Press release]. Retrieved from www.cdc.gov/media/releases/2018
/p0607-suicide-prevention.html

Floman, J. L., Brackett, M. A., Schmitt, L., & Baron, W. (2018, May). School climate, teacher affect, and teacher well-being: Direct and indirect effects. Presented
at the Association for Psychological Science Convention in San Francisco, CA.

Gallup Inc. (2014). State of America's schools: The path to winning again in education. Retrieved from www.gallup.com/services/178709/state-america-schools
-report.aspx

Goleman, D. (1997). *Emotional Intelligence: Why It Can Matter More Than IQ*. New
York: Bantam Books.

Lipson, S. K., Lattie, E. G., & Eisenberg, D. (2018). Increased rates of mental health
service utilization by US college students: 10-year population-level trends (2007–
2017). *Psychiatric Services, 70*(1), 60–63. doi.org/10.1176/appi.ps.201800332

Moeller, J., Ivcevic, Z., Brackett, M. A., & White, A. E. (2018). Mixed emotions:
Network analyses of intra-individual co-occurrences within and across situations.
Emotion, 18(8), 1106–1121. doi.org/10.1037/emo0000419

Moeller, J., Brackett, M., Ivcevic, Z., & White, A. (under review). High school students' feelings: Discoveries from a large national survey and an experience sam-
pling study. *Learning and Instruction.*

Salovey, P., & Mayer, J. D. (1990). Emotional intelligence. *Imagination, Cognition
and Personality, 9*(3), 185–211. doi.org/10.2190/DUGG-P24E-52WK-6CDG

Steinberg, L. (2014). *Age of Opportunity: Lessons from the New Science of Adolescence.*
New York: Houghton Mifflin Harcourt.

UNICEF. (2013). Child well-being in rich countries: A comparative overview, innocenti
report card 11. Florence: UNICEF Office of Research. Retrieved from www
.unicef-irc.org/publications/pdf/rc11_eng.pdf

2. Emotions Are Information

Aldao, A., Nolen-Hoeksema, S., & Schweizer, S. (2010). Emotion-regulation strategies across psychopathology: A meta-analytic review. *Clinical Psychology Review,
30*(2), 217–237. doi:10.1016/j.cpr.2009.11.004

Amabile, T. M., Barsade, S. G., Mueller, J. S., & Staw, B. M. (2005). Affect and creativity at work. *Administrative Science Quarterly, 50*(3), 367–403. doi.org/10.2189/asqu.2005.50.3.367

Anderson, N., De Dreu, C. K., & Nijstad, B. A. (2004). The routinization of innovation research: A constructively critical review of the state-of-the-science. *Journal of Organizational Behavior, 25*(2), 147–173.

Appleton, A. A., Holdsworth, E., Ryan, M., & Tracy, M. (2017). Measuring childhood adversity in life course cardiovascular research: A systematic review. *Psychosomatic Medicine, 79*(4), 434–440.

Aristotle. (1984). *The Complete Works of Aristotle: The Revised Oxford Translation.* J. Barnes (Ed.). Princeton, NJ: Princeton University Press.

Aschbacher, K., O'Donovan, A., Wolkowitz, O. M., Dhabhar, F. S., Su, Y., & Epel, E. (2013). Good stress, bad stress and oxidative stress: Insights from anticipatory cortisol reactivity. *Psychoneuroendocrinology, 38*(9), 1698–1708.

Baas, M., De Dreu, C. K., & Nijstad, B. A. (2008). A meta-analysis of 25 years of mood-creativity research: Hedonic tone, activation, or regulatory focus? *Psychological Bulletin, 134*(6), 779–806. doi.org/10.1037/a0012815

Bal, E., Harden, E., Lamb, D., Van Hecke, A. V., Denver, J. W., & Porges, S. W. (2010). Emotion recognition in children with autism spectrum disorders: Relations to eye gaze and autonomic state. *Journal of Autism and Developmental Disorders, 40*(3), 358–370.

Barrett, L. F. (2017). *How Emotions Are Made: The Secret Life of the Brain.* Boston: Houghton Mifflin Harcourt.

Barrett, L. F., Mesquita, B., Ochsner, K. N., & Gross, J. J. (2007). The experience of emotion. *Annual Review of Psychology, 58*, 373–403. doi.org/10.1146/annurev.psych.58.110405.085709

Barsade, S. G., & Gibson, D. E. (2007). Why does affect matter in organizations? *Academy of Management Perspectives, 21*(1), 36–59. doi.org/10.5465/amp.2007.24286163

Batson, C. D. (2011). *Altruism in Humans.* Oxford: Oxford University Press.

Bennett, M. P., & Lengacher, C. (2008). Humor and laughter may influence health: III. Laughter and health outcomes. *Evidence-Based Complementary and Alternative Medicine, 5*(1), 37–40.

Berna, C., Leknes, S., Holmes, E. A., Edwards, R. R., Goodwin, G. M., & Tracey, I. (2010). Induction of depressed mood disrupts emotion regulation neurocircuitry and enhances pain unpleasantness. *Biological Psychiatry, 67*(11), 1083–1090.

Berridge, K. C. (2007). The debate over dopamine's role in reward: The case for incentive salience. *Psychopharmacology, 191*(3), 391–431. doi.org/10.1007/s00213-006-0578-x

Blair, C., & Raver, C. C. (2016). Poverty, stress, and brain development: New directions for prevention and intervention. *Academic Pediatrics, 16*(3), S30–S36. doi.org/10.1016/j.acap.2016.01.010

Bodenhausen, G. V., Sheppard, L. A., & Kramer, G. P. (1994). Negative affect and social judgment: The differential impact of anger and sadness. *European Journal of Social Psychology, 24*(1), 45–62.

Boekaerts, M. (2010). The crucial role of motivation and emotion in classroom learning. In H. Dumont, D. Istance, & F. Benavides (Eds.), *The Nature of Learning: Using Research to Inspire Practice* (pp. 91–111). Paris: OECD.

Bower, G. H. (1981). Mood and memory. *American Psychologist, 36*(2), 129–148. doi.org/10.1037/0003-066X.36.2.129

Bower, G. H. (1992). How might emotions affect learning. In S. Christianson (Ed.), *The Handbook of Emotion and Memory: Research and Theory* (pp. 3–31). Oxford: Psychology Press.

Bower, G. H., & Forgas, J. P. (2001). Mood and social memory. In J. P. Forgas (Ed.), *The Handbook of Affect and Social Cognition* (pp. 95–120). Mahwah, NJ: Erlbaum.

Bowers, T. (2004). Stress, teaching and teacher health. *Education 3–13: International Journal of Primary, Elementary and Early Years Education, 32*, 73–80. doi.org/10.1080/03004270485200361

Brackett, M. A., Floman, J. L., Ashton-James, C., Cherkasskiy, L., & Salovey, P. (2013). The influence of teacher emotion on grading practices: A preliminary look at the evaluation of student writing. *Teachers and Teaching, 19*(6), 634–646.

Brackett, M. A., Rivers, S. E., & Salovey, P. (2011). Emotional intelligence: Implications for personal, social, academic, and workplace success. *Social and Personality Psychology Compass, 5*(1), 88–103. doi.org/10.1111/j.1751-9004.2010.00334.x

Bradley, M. M., & Lang, P. J. (2000). Emotion and motivation. In J. T. Cacioppo, L. G. Tassinary, & G. G. Berntson (Eds.), *Handbook of Psychophysiology* (pp. 602–642). Cambridge: Cambridge University Press.

Brooks, J. L. (Producer & Director). (1987). *Broadcast News*. [Film]. USA: Twentieth Century Fox.

Burgdorf, J., & Panksepp, J. (2006). The neurobiology of positive emotions. *Neuroscience & Biobehavioral Reviews, 30*(2), 173–187. doi.org/10.1016/j.neubiorev.2005.06.001

Cantor, N., & Kihlstrom, J. F. (2000). Social intelligence. In R. J. Sternberg & S. B. Kaufman (Eds.), *Handbook of Intelligence* (pp. 359–379). Cambridge: Cambridge University Press.

Chida, Y., & Steptoe, A. (2009). The association of anger and hostility with future coronary heart disease: A meta-analytic review of prospective evidence. *Journal of the American College of Cardiology, 53*(11), 936–946.

Christianson, S. A. (2014). *The Handbook of Emotion and Memory: Research and Theory*. Oxford: Psychology Press.

Cohen, T. R., Panter, A. T., & Turan, N. (2012). Guilt proneness and moral character. *Current Directions in Psychological Science, 21*(5), 355–359. doi.org/10.1177/0963721412454874

Cosmides, L., & Tooby, J. (2000). Evolutionary psychology and the emotions. In M. Lewis & J. M. Haviland-Jones (Eds.), *Handbook of Emotions* (pp. 91–115). New York: Guilford Publications.

Côté, S., & Miners, C. T. (2006). Emotional intelligence, cognitive intelligence, and job performance. *Administrative Science Quarterly, 51*(1), 1–28. doi.org/10.2189/asqu.51.1.1

Cozolino, L. (2014). *The Neuroscience of Human Relationships: Attachment and the Developing Social Brain*. New York: W. W. Norton & Company.

Crum, A. J., Akinola, M., Martin, A., & Fath, S. (2017). The role of stress mindset in shaping cognitive, emotional, and physiological responses to challenging and threatening stress. *Anxiety, Stress, & Coping, 30*(4), 379–395.

Crum, A. J., Salovey, P., & Achor, S. (2013). Rethinking stress: The role of mindsets in determining the stress response. *Journal of Personality and Social Psychology, 104*(4), 716–733.

Damasio, A. R. (1995). *Descartes' Error*. New York: Random House.

Darr, W., & Johns, G. (2008). Work strain, health and absenteeism: A meta-analysis. *Journal of Occupational Health Psychology, 13*, 293–318. doi.org/10.1037/a0012639

Darwin, C. (1872/1998). *The Expression of the Emotions in Man and Animals*. Oxford: Oxford University Press.

Dave, N. D., Xiang, L., Rehm, K. E., & Marshall, G. D. (2011). Stress and allergic diseases. *Immunology and Allergy Clinics, 31*(1), 55–68.

Davidson, R. J., & Begley, S. (2012). *The Emotional Life of Your Brain: How its unique patterns affect the way you think, feel, and live—and how you can change them*. London: Penguin.

Deci, E. L., & Ryan, R. M. (2008). Self-determination theory: A macrotheory of human motivation, development, and health. *Canadian Psychology/Psychologie Canadienne, 49*(3), 182–185.

DeLongis, A., Folkman, S., & Lazarus, R. S. (1988). The impact of daily stress on health and mood: Psychological and social resources as mediators. *Journal of Personality and Social Psychology, 54*(3), 486–495.

Denson, T. F., Spanovic, M., & Miller, N. (2009). Cognitive appraisals and emotions predict cortisol and immune responses: A meta-analysis of acute laboratory social stressors and emotion inductions. *Psychological Bulletin, 135*(6), 823–853.

DeSteno, D., Gross, J. J., & Kubzansky, L. (2013). Affective science and health: The

importance of emotion and emotion regulation. *Health Psychology, 32*(5), 474. doi
.org/10.1037/a0030259

Dhabhar, F. S. (2014). Effects of stress on immune function: The good, the bad, and
the beautiful. *Immunologic Research, 58*(2–3), 193–210.

Dunbar, R. I. (1998). The social brain hypothesis. *Evolutionary Anthropology: Issues,
News, and Reviews, 6*(5), 178–190.

Durlak, J. A., Weissberg, R. P., Dymnicki, A. B., Taylor, R. D., & Schellinger, K. B.
(2011). The impact of enhancing students' social and emotional learning: A meta-
analysis of school-based universal interventions. *Child Development, 82*(1), 405–
432. doi.org/10.1111/j.1467-8624.2010.01564.x

Ekman, P. (1992). An argument for basic emotions. *Cognition & Emotion, 6*(3–4),
169–200. doi.org/10.1080/02699939208411068

Ekman, P. E., & Davidson, R. J. (1994). *The Nature of Emotion: Fundamental Questions*. Oxford: Oxford University Press.

Elzinga, B. M., & Roelofs, K. (2005). Cortisol-induced impairments of working
memory require acute sympathetic activation. *Behavioral Neuroscience, 119*(1),
98–103. doi.org/10.1037/0735-7044.119.1.98

Emanuele, E., Politi, P., Bianchi, M., Minoretti, P., Bertona, M., & Geroldi, D.
(2006). Raised plasma nerve growth factor levels associated with early-stage romantic love. *Psychoneuroendocrinology, 31*(3), 288–294.

Epel, E., Prather, A. A., Puterman, E., & Tomiyama, A. J. (2016). Eat, drink, and be
sedentary: A review of health behaviors' effects on emotions and affective states,
and implications for interventions. In L. F. Barrett, M. Lewis, & J. M. Haviland-
Jones (Eds.), *Handbook of Emotions* (pp. 685–706). New York: Guilford Publications.

Fischer, A. H. & Manstead, A. S. R. (2016). Social functions or emotion and emotion
regulation. In L. F. Barrett, M. Lewis, & J. M. Haviland-Jones (Eds.), *Handbook
of Emotions* (pp. 424–439). New York: Guilford Publications.

Floman, J. L., Brackett, M.A., Schmitt, L., & Baron, W. (2018, May). School climate, teacher affect, and teacher well-being: Direct and indirect effects. Presented
at the Association for Psychological Science Convention in San Francisco, CA.

Forgas, J. P. (1998). On being happy and mistaken: Mood effects on the fundamental
attribution error. *Journal of Personality and Social Psychology, 75*(2), 318–331.

Forgas, J. P. (2011). Can negative affect eliminate the power of first impressions? Affective influences on primacy and recency effects in impression formation. *Journal
of Experimental Social Psychology, 47*(2), 425–429.

Forgas, J. P. (2013). Don't worry, be sad! On the cognitive, motivational, and interpersonal benefits of negative mood. *Current Directions in Psychological Science,
22*(3), 225–232.

Forgas, J. P. (2014). On the regulatory functions of mood: Affective influences on memory, judgments and behavior. In J. P. Forgas & E. Harmon-Jones (Eds.), *Motivation and its Regulation: The Control Within*, (pp. 169–192). New York: Psychology Press.

Forgas, J. P., & East, R. (2008). On being happy and gullible: Mood effects on skepticism and the detection of deception. *Journal of Experimental Social Psychology*, *44*(5), 1362–1367.

Forgas, J. P., & George, J. M. (2001). Affective influences on judgments and behavior in organizations: An information processing perspective. *Organizational Behavior and Human Decision Processes*, *86*(1), 3–34. doi.org/10.1006/obhd.2001.2971

Fowler, J. H., & Christakis, N. A. (2008). Dynamic spread of happiness in a large social network: Longitudinal analysis over 20 years in the Framingham Heart Study. *BMJ*, *337*, a2338.

Fredrickson, B. L. (1998). What good are positive emotions? *Review of General Psychology*, *2*(3), 300–319.

Fredrickson, B. L. (2013). Positive emotions broaden and build. In P. Devine & A. Plant (Eds.), *Advances in Experimental Social Psychology* (vol. 47, pp. 1–53). Cambridge, MA: Academic Press.

Fredrickson, B. L., & Branigan, C. (2005). Positive emotions broaden the scope of attention and thought-action repertoires. *Cognition & Emotion*, *19*(3), 313–332. doi.org/10.1080/02699930441000238

Fredrickson, B. L., Tugade, M. M., Waugh, C. E., & Larkin, G. R. (2003). What good are positive emotions in crisis? A prospective study of resilience and emotions following the terrorist attacks on the United States on September 11th, 2001. *Journal of Personality and Social Psychology*, *84*(2), 365–376.

Frevert, U. (2016). The history of emotions. In L. F. Barrett, M. Lewis, & J. M. Haviland-Jones (Eds.), *Handbook of Emotions* (pp. 49–65). New York: Guilford Publications.

Gardner, H. (1992). *Multiple intelligences* (vol. 5, p. 56). Minnesota Center for Arts Education.

Goetz, J. L., Keltner, D., & Simon-Thomas, E. (2010). Compassion: An evolutionary analysis and empirical review. *Psychological Bulletin*, *136*(3), 351–374.

Goetzmann, W. N., Kim, D., Kumar, A., & Wang, Q. (2014). Weather-induced mood, institutional investors, and stock returns. *Review of Financial Studies*, *28*(1), 73–111.

Goleman, D. (1995). *Emotional Intelligence: Why It Can Matter More Than IQ*. New York: Bantam Books.

Greenberg, M. T., Brown, J. L., & Abenavoli, R. M. (2016, September). *Teacher stress and health: Effects on teachers, students, and schools*. Edna Bennett Pierce Prevention

Research Center, Pennsylvania State University. Retrieved from www.rwjf.org/en/library/research/2016/07/teacher-stress-and-health.html

Gross, J. J. (2002). Emotion regulation: Affective, cognitive, and social consequences. *Psychophysiology, 39*(3), 281–291. doi.org/10.1017/S0048577201393198

Guhn, M., Schonert-Reichl, K. A., Gadermann, A. M., Hymel, S., & Hertzman, C. (2013). A population study of victimization, relationships, and well-being in middle childhood. *Journal of Happiness Studies, 14*(5), 1529–1541.

Guilford, J. P. (1967). *The Nature of Human Intelligence.* New York: McGraw-Hill.

Haidt, J. (2001). The emotional dog and its rational tail: A social intuitionist approach to moral judgment. *Psychological Review, 108*(4), 814–834. doi.org/10.1017/CBO9780511814273.055

Haidt, J. (2012). *The Righteous Mind: Why Good People Are Divided by Politics and Religion.* New York: Vintage.

Hajcak, G., Jackson, F., Ferri, J., & Weinberg, A. (2016). Emotion and attention. In L. F. Barrett, M. Lewis, & J. M. Haviland-Jones (Eds.), *Handbook of Emotions* (pp. 595–612). New York: Guilford Publications.

Hargreaves, A. (1998). The emotional practice of teaching. *Teaching and Teacher Education, 14*(8), 835–854. doi.org/10.1016/S0742-051X(98)00025-0

Hascher, T. (2010). Learning and emotion: Perspectives for theory and research. *European Educational Research Journal, 9*(1), 13–28. doi.org/10.2304/eerj.2010.9.1.13

Hawkley, L. C., & Cacioppo, J. T. (2010). Loneliness matters: A theoretical and empirical review of consequences and mechanisms. *Annals of Behavioral Medicine, 40*(2), 218–227.

Hirshleifer, D., & Shumway, T. (2003). Good day sunshine: Stock returns and the weather. *Journal of Finance, 58*(3), 1009–1032.

Huntsinger, J. R. (2013). Does emotion directly tune the scope of attention? *Current Directions in Psychological Science, 22*(4), 265–270. doi.org/10.1177/0963721413480364

Huntsinger, J. R., Isbell, L. M., & Clore, G. L. (2014). The affective control of thought: Malleable, not fixed. *Psychological Review, 121*(4), 600–618. doi.org/10.1037/a0037669

Hutcherson, C. A., & Gross, J. J. (2011). The moral emotions: A social-functionalist account of anger, disgust, and contempt. *Journal of Personality and Social Psychology, 100*(4), 719–737. doi.org/10.1037/a0022408

IBM. (2010, May 18). IBM 2010 global CEO study: Creativity selected as most crucial factor for future success. Retrieved from www-03.ibm.com/press/us/en/pressrelease/31670.wss

Innes-Ker, Å., & Niedenthal, P. M. (2002). Emotion concepts and emotional states in social judgment and categorization. *Journal of Personality and Social Psychology,* *83*(4), 804–816.

Isbell, L. M., & Lair, E. C. (2013). Moods, emotions, and evaluations as information. In D. Carlston (Ed.), *Handbook of Social Cognition* (pp. 435–462). Oxford: Oxford University Press.

Isen, A. M. (1999). On the relationship between affect and creative problem solving. In S. W. Russ (Ed.), *Affect, Creative Experience, and Psychological Adjustment* (pp. 3–17). Oxfordshire, UK: Taylor & Francis.

Isen, A. M., Daubman, K. A., & Nowicki, G. P. (1987). Positive affect facilitates creative problem solving. *Journal of Personality and Social Psychology, 52*(6), 1122–1131. doi.org/10.1037//0022-3514.52.6.1122

Isen, A. M., Niedenthal, P. M., & Cantor, N. (1992). An influence of positive affect on social categorization. *Motivation and Emotion, 16*(1), 65–78.

Ivcevic, Z., Bazhydai, M., Hoffmann, J., & Brackett, M. A. (2017). Creativity in the domain of emotions. In J. C. Kaufman, V. P. Glaveanu, & J. Baer (Eds.), *Cambridge Handbook of Creativity Across Different Domains* (Pp. 525–549). Cambridge: Cambridge University Press.

Ivcevic, Z., Brackett, M. A., & Mayer, J. D. (2007). Emotional intelligence and emotional creativity. *Journal of Personality, 75*(2), 199–236.

John, A., Glendenning, A. C., Marchant, A., Montgomery, P., Stewart, A., Wood, S., . . . Hawton, K. (2018). Self-harm, suicidal behaviours, and cyberbullying in children and young people: Systematic review. *Journal of Medical Internet Research, 20*(4), e129.

Kabat-Zinn, J. (1990). *Full Catastrophe Living: Using the wisdom of your body and mind to face stress, pain, and illness.* New York: Delta.

Kahneman, D., (2011). *Thinking, Fast and Slow.* New York: Farrar, Straus and Giroux.

Keltner, D. (2019). Toward a consensual taxonomy of emotions. *Cognition and Emotion, 33*(1), 1–6. doi.org/10.1080/02699931.2019.1574397

Keltner, D., & Gross, J. J. (1999). Functional accounts of emotions. *Cognition and Emotion, 13*(5), 467–480. doi.org/10.1080/026999399379140

Keltner, D., & Haidt, J. (1999). Social functions of emotions at four levels of analysis. *Cognition and Emotion, 13*(5), 505–521. doi.org/10.1080/026999399379168

Keltner, D., & Kring, A. M. (1998). Emotion, social function, and psychopathology. *Review of General Psychology, 2*(3), 320–342.

Keltner, D., Ellsworth, P. C., & Edwards, K. (1993). Beyond simple pessimism: Effects of sadness and anger on social perception. *Journal of Personality and Social Psychology, 64*(5), 740–752.

Kemp, A. H., Gray, M. A., Silberstein, R. B., Armstrong, S. M., & Nathan, P. J. (2004). Augmentation of serotonin enhances pleasant and suppresses unpleasant cortical electrophysiological responses to visual emotional stimuli in humans. *Neuroimage, 22*(3), 1084–1096. doi.org/10.1016/j.neuroimage.2004.03.022

Kensinger, E. A. & Schacter, D. L. (2016). Memory and emotion. In L. F. Barrett, M. Lewis, & J. M. Haviland-Jones (Eds.), *Handbook of Emotions* (pp. 564–578). New York: Guilford Publications.

Kiecolt-Glaser, J. K., McGuire, L., Robles, T. F., & Glaser, R. (2002). Emotions, morbidity, and mortality: New perspectives from psychoneuroimmunology. *Annual Review of Psychology, 53*(1), 83–107.

Kim, K. H., Cramond, B., & VanTassel-Baska, J. (2010). The relationship between creativity and intelligence. In J. C. Kaufman, & R. J. Sternberg (Eds.), *The Cambridge Handbook of Creativity* (pp. 395–412). New York: Cambridge University Press.

Kubzansky, L. D., & Kawachi, I. (2000). Going to the heart of the matter: Do negative emotions cause coronary heart disease? *Journal of Psychosomatic Research, 48*(4–5), 323–337. doi.org/10.1016/S0022-3999(99)00091-4

Kubzansky, L. D., Huffman, J. C., Boehm, J. K., Hernandez, R., Kim, E. S., Koga, H. K., . . . Labarthe, D. R. (2018). Positive psychological well-being and cardiovascular disease: JACC health promotion series. *Journal of the American College of Cardiology, 72*(12), 1382–1396. doi.org/10.1016/j.jacc.2018.07.042

LeDoux, J. (1997). The emotional brain: The mysterious underpinnings of emotional life. *World and I, 12,* 281–285.

Lempert, K. M. & Phelps, E. A. (2016). Affect in economic decision making. In L. F. Barrett, M. Lewis, & J. M. Haviland-Jones (Eds.), *Handbook of Emotions* (pp. 98–112). New York: Guilford Publications.

Lerner, J. S., Li, Y., Valdesolo, P., & Kassam, K. S. (2015). Emotion and decision making. *Annual Review of Psychology, 66,* 799–823. doi.org/10.1146/annurev-psych-010213-115043

Lerner, J. S., Small, D. A., & Loewenstein, G. (2004). Heart strings and purse strings: Carryover effects of emotions on economic decisions. *Psychological Science, 15*(5), 337–341.

Lewis, M. (2016). The emergence of human emotions. In L. F. Barrett, M. Lewis, & J. M. Haviland-Jones (Eds.), *Handbook of Emotions* (pp. 272–292). New York: Guilford Publications.

Lopes, P. N., Salovey, P., Côté, S., Beers, M., & Petty, R. E. (2005). Emotion regulation abilities and the quality of social interaction. *Emotion, 5*(1), 113–118. doi.org/10.1037/1528-3542.5.1.113

Lumley, M. A., Cohen, J. L., Borszcz, G. S., Cano, A., Radcliffe, A. M., Porter, L. S., . . . Keefe, F. J. (2011). Pain and emotion: A biopsychosocial review of recent research. *Journal of Clinical Psychology, 67*(9), 942–968.

Lupien, S. J., McEwen, B. S., Gunnar, M. R., & Heim, C. (2009). Effects of stress throughout the lifespan on the brain, behaviour and cognition. *Nature Reviews Neuroscience, 10,* 434–445. doi.org/10.1038/nrn2639

Lyubomirsky, S., & Lepper, H. S. (1999). A measure of subjective happiness: Preliminary reliability and construct validation. *Social Indicators Research, 46*(2), 137–155. doi.org/10.1023/A:1006824100041

Lyubomirsky, S., King, L., & Diener, E. (2005). The benefits of frequent positive affect: Does happiness lead to success? *Psychological Bulletin, 131*(6), 803–855. doi.org/10.1037/0033-2909.131.6.803

Mackintosh, N., & Mackintosh, N. J. (2011). *IQ and Human Intelligence.* Oxford: Oxford University Press.

Martin, R. A., & Ford, T. (2018). *The Psychology of Humor: An Integrative Approach.* Cambridge, MA: Academic Press.

Mayer, J. D., Caruso, D. R., & Salovey, P. (2016). The ability model of emotional intelligence: Principles and updates. *Emotion Review, 8*(4), 290–300. doi.org/10.1177/1754073916639667

Mayer, J. D., Gaschke, Y. N., Braverman, D. L., & Evans, T. W. (1992). Mood-congruent judgment is a general effect. *Journal of Personality and Social Psychology, 63*(1), 119–132. doi.org/10.1037/0022-3514.63.1.119

Mayer, J. D., McCormick, L. J., & Strong, S. E. (1995). Mood-congruent memory and natural mood: New evidence. *Personality and Social Psychology Bulletin, 21*(7), 736–46. doi.org/10.1177/0146167295217008

Mayer, J. D., Salovey, P., & Caruso, D. R. (2008). Emotional intelligence: New ability or eclectic traits? *American Psychologist, 63*(6), 503–517. doi.org/10.1037/0003-066X.63.6.503

McCrae, R. R. (1987). Creativity, divergent thinking, and openness to experience. *Journal of Personality and Social Psychology, 52*(6), 1258–1265. doi.org/10.1037/0022-3514.52.6.1258

McCraty, R., & Childre, D. (2004). The grateful heart: The psychophysiology of appreciation. In R. A. Emmons & M. E. McCullough (Eds.), *The Psychology of Gratitude* (p. 230). Oxford: Oxford University Press.

McEwen, B. S., Bowles, N. P., Gray, J. D., Hill, M. N., Hunter, R. G., Karatsoreos, I. N., & Nasca, C. (2015). Mechanisms of stress in the brain. *Nature Neuroscience, 18*(10), 1353–1363. doi.org/10.1038/nn.4086

McGonigal, K. (2016). *The Upside of Stress: Why stress is good for you, and how to get good at it.* London, England: Penguin.

McIntyre, T., McIntyre, S., & Francis, D. (2017). *Educator Stress.* New York: Springer.

Moeller, J., Ivcevic, Z., Brackett, M. A., & White, A. E. (2018). Mixed emotions: Network analyses of intra-individual co-occurrences within and across situations. *Emotion, 18*(8), 1106–1121.

Moore, S. E., Norman, R. E., Suetani, S., Thomas, H. J., Sly, P. D., & Scott, J. G. (2017). Consequences of bullying victimization in childhood and adolescence: A systematic review and meta-analysis. *World Journal of Psychiatry, 7*(1), 60–76.

Niedenthal, P. M., Mermillod, M., Maringer, M., & Hess, U. (2010). The simulation of smiles (SIMS) model: Embodied simulation and the meaning of facial expression. *Behavioral and Brain Sciences, 33*(6), 417–433.

Nowak, M. A. (2006). Five rules for the evolution of cooperation. *Science, 314*(5805), 1560–1563.

Nusbaum, E. C., & Silvia, P. J. (2011). Are intelligence and creativity really so different? Fluid intelligence, executive processes, and strategy use in divergent thinking. *Intelligence, 39*(1), 36–45.

Oatley, K., Keltner, D., & Jenkins, J. M. (2018). *Understanding Emotions*. Hoboken, NJ: Blackwell Publishing.

Öhman, A., Flykt, A., & Esteves, F. (2001). Emotion drives attention: Detecting the snake in the grass. *Journal of Experimental Psychology: General, 130*(3), 466–478. doi:10.1037/AXJ96-3445.130.3.466

Oveis, C., Horberg, E. J., & Keltner, D. (2010). Compassion, pride, and social intuitions of self-other similarity. *Journal of Personality and Social Psychology, 98*(4), 618–630.

Panksepp, J. (2009). Brain emotional systems and qualities of mental life: From animal models of affect to implications for psychotherapeutics. In D. Fosha, D. J. Siegel, & M. F. Solomon (Eds.), *The Healing Power of Emotion: Affective Neuroscience, Development & Clinical Practice* (pp. 1–26). New York: W. W. Norton & Company.

Pekrun, R., & Linnenbrink-Garcia, L. (2012). Academic emotions and student engagement. In S. Christenson & A. Reschly, & C. Wylie (Eds.), *Handbook of Research on Student Engagement* (pp. 259–282). Boston, MA: Springer.

Phelps, E. A. (2004). Human emotion and memory: Interactions of the amygdala and hippocampal complex. *Current Opinion in Neurobiology, 14*(2), 198–202. doi.org/10.1016/j.conb.2004.03.015

Psychologies. (2011, August 24). The link between emotions and health. Retrieved from www.psychologies.co.uk/self/the-link-between-emotions-and-health.html

Raven, J. C., & Court, J. H. (1998). *Raven's Progressive Matrices and Vocabulary Scales*. Oxford: Oxford Pyschologists Press.

Redelmeier, D. A., & Baxter, S. D. (2009). Rainy weather and medical school admission interviews. *Canadian Medical Association Journal, 181*(12), 933.

Redwine, L., Henry, B. L., Pung, M. A., Wilson, K., Chinh, K., Knight, B., . . . Mills, P. J. (2016). A pilot randomized study of a gratitude journaling intervention on HRV and inflammatory biomarkers in Stage B heart failure patients. *Psychosomatic Medicine, 78*(6), 667–676.

Rook, K. S. (2001). Emotional health and positive versus negative social exchanges: A daily diary analysis. *Applied Developmental Science, 5*(2), 86–97.

Roorda, D. L., Koomen, H. M., Spilt, J. L., & Oort, F. J. (2011). The influence of affective teacher–student relationships on students' school engagement and achievement: A meta-analytic approach. *Review of Educational Research, 81*(4), 493–529. doi.org/10.3102/0034654311421793

Roseman, I. J. (2013). Appraisal in the emotion system: Coherence in strategies for coping. *Emotion Review, 5*(2), 141–149. doi.org/10.1177/1754073912469591

Salim, S., Asghar, M., Chugh, G., Taneja, M., Xia, Z., & Saha, K. (2010). Oxidative stress: A potential recipe for anxiety, hypertension and insulin resistance. *Brain Research, 1359*, 178–185.

Salovey, P., & Mayer, J. D. (1990). Emotional intelligence. *Imagination, Cognition and Personality, 9*(3), 185–211. doi.org/10.2190/DUGG-P24E-52WK-6CDG

Salovey, P., Rothman, A. J., Detweiler, J. B., & Steward, W. T. (2000). Emotional states and physical health. *American Psychologist, 55*(1), 110–121.

Sands, M., Ngo, N., & Isaacowitz, D. M. (2016). The interplay of motivation and emotion: View from adulthood and old age. In L. F. Barrett, M. Lewis, & J. M. Haviland-Jones (Eds.), *Handbook of Emotions* (pp. 336–349). New York: Guilford Publications.

Sapolsky, R. M. (2015). Stress and the brain: Individual variability and the inverted-U. *Nature Neuroscience, 18*(10), 1344–1346.

Sbarra, D. A., & Coan, J. A. (2018). Relationships and health: The critical role of affective science. *Emotion Review, 10*(1), 40–54. doi.org/10.1177/1754073917696584

Scarantino, A. (2016). The philosophy of emotions and its impact on affective science. In L. F. Barrett, M. Lewis, & J. M. Haviland-Jones (Eds.), *Handbook of Emotions* (pp. 3–48). New York: Guilford Publications.

Schmeichel, B. J., & Inzlicht, M. (2013). Incidental and integral effects of emotions on self-control. In M. D. Robinson, E. R. Watkins, & E. Harmon-Jones (Eds.), *Handbook of Cognition and Emotion* (pp. 272–290). New York: Guilford Publications.

Schonert-Reichl, K. A., Guhn, M., Gadermann, A. M., Hymel, S., Sweiss, L., & Hertzman, C. (2013). Development and validation of the Middle Years Development Instrument (MDI): Assessing children's well-being and assets across multiple contexts. *Social Indicators Research, 114*(2), 345–369.

Schupp, H. T., Flaisch, T., Stockburger, J., & Junghöfer, M. (2006). Emotion and attention: Event-related brain potential studies. *Progress in Brain Research, 156*, 31–51. doi.org/10.1016/S0079-6123(06)56002-9

Schutz, P. A., Pekrun, R., & Phye, G. D. (2007). *Emotion in education* (vol. 10). P. A. Schutz & R. Pekrun (Eds.). San Diego, CA: Academic Press.

Schwarz, N., & Clore, G. L. (1983). Mood, misattribution, and judgments of well-being: Informative and directive functions of affective states. *Journal of Personality and Social Psychology, 45*(3), 513–523. doi.org/10.1037/0022-3514.45.3.513

Schwarz, N., & Clore, G. L. (2003). Mood as information: 20 years later. *Psychological Inquiry, 14*(3–4), 296–303. doi.org/10.1080/1047840X.2003.9682896

Schwarz, N., & Clore, G. L. (2007). Feelings and phenomenal experiences. In A. W. Kruglanski & E. T. Higgins (Eds.), *Social Psychology: Handbook of Basic Principles* (pp. 385–407). New York: Guilford Press.

Selye, H. (2013). *Stress in Health and Disease.* Waltham, MA: Butterworth-Heinemann.

Selye, H., Memedovic, S., Grisham, J. R., Denson, T. F., & Moulds, M. L. (2010). The effects of trait reappraisal and suppression on anger and blood pressure in response to provocation. *Journal of Research in Personality, 44*(4), 540–543.

Sharma, S. (2016). Life events stress, emotional vital signs and hypertension. In A. K. Dalal & G. Misra (Eds.), *New Directions in Health Psychology* (pp. 389–408). New Delhi, India: Sage Publications.

Shields, G. S., Sazma, M. A., & Yonelinas, A. P. (2016). The effects of acute stress on core executive functions: A meta-analysis and comparison with cortisol. *Neuroscience & Biobehavioral Reviews, 68*, 651–668. doi.org/10.1016/j.neubiorev.2016.06.038

Shiota, M. N., Campos, B., Oveis, C., Hertenstein, M. J., Simon-Thomas, E., & Keltner, D. (2017). Beyond happiness: Building a science of discrete positive emotions. *American Psychologist, 72*(7), 617–643. doi.org/10.1037/a0040456

Shonkoff, J., Levitt, P., Bunge, S., Cameron, J., Duncan, G., Fisher, P., & Nox, N. (2015). Supportive relationships and active skill-building strengthen the foundations of resilience: Working paper 13. Cambridge, UK: National Scientific Council on the Developing Child.

Silvia, P. J., & Beaty, R. E. (2012). Making creative metaphors: The importance of fluid intelligence for creative thought. *Intelligence, 40*(4), 343–351.

Silvia, P. J., Martin, C., & Nusbaum, E. C. (2009). A snapshot of creativity: Evaluating a quick and simple method for assessing divergent thinking. *Thinking Skills and Creativity, 4*(2), 79–85. doi.org/10.1016/j.tsc.2009.06.005

Sinclair, R. C., & Mark, M. M. (1992). The influence of mood state on judgment and action: Effects on persuasion, categorization, social justice, person perception, and judgmental accuracy. In L. L. Martin & A. Tesser (Eds.), *The Construction of Social Judgments* (pp. 165–193). Hillsdale, NJ: Lawrence Erlbaum Associates, Inc.

Singer, J. A., & Salovey, P. (2010). *Remembered Self: Emotion and Memory in Personality.* New York: Simon & Schuster.

Stefanucci, J. K., Gagnon, K. T., & Lessard, D. A. (2011). Follow your heart: Emotion adaptively influences perception. *Social and Personality Psychology Compass, 5*(6), 296–308.

Steinberg, L. (2005). Cognitive and affective development in adolescence. *Trends in Cognitive Sciences, 9*(2), 69–74. doi.org/10.1016/j.tics.2004.12.005

Sternberg, R. J. (1999). The theory of successful intelligence. *Review of General Psychology, 3*(4), 292–316. doi.org/10.1037/1089-2680.3.4.292

Sy, T., & Côté, S. (2004). Emotional intelligence: A key ability to succeed in the matrix organization. *Journal of Management Development, 23*(5), 437–455. doi.org/10.1108/02621710410537056

Tamir, M., Mitchell, C., & Gross, J. J. (2008). Hedonic and instrumental motives in anger regulation. *Psychological Science, 19*(4), 324–328.

Tan, H. B., & Forgas, J. P. (2010). When happiness makes us selfish, but sadness makes us fair: Affective influences on interpersonal strategies in the dictator game. *Journal of Experimental Social Psychology, 46*(3), 571–576.

Tangney, J. P., Stuewig, J., & Mashek, D. J. (2007). Moral emotions and moral behavior. *Annual Review of Psychology, 58*, 345–372. doi.org/10.1146/annurev.psych.56.091103.070145

Tarullo, A. R., & Gunnar, M. R. (2006). Child maltreatment and the developing HPA axis. *Hormones and Behavior, 50*(4), 632–639.

Thorndike, E. L. (1920). Intelligence and its uses. *Harper's Magazine*, 140, 227–235.

Torrance, E. P. (1988). The nature of creativity as manifest in its testing. In R. J. Sternberg (Ed.), *The Nature of Creativity: Contemporary Psychological Perspectives* (pp. 43–75). Cambridge: Cambridge University Press.

Tversky, A., & Kahneman, D. (1974). Judgment under uncertainty: Heuristics and biases. *Science, 185*(4157), 1124–1131.

Van Kleef, G. A., Anastasopoulou, C., & Nijstad, B. A. (2010). Can expressions of anger enhance creativity? A test of the emotions as social information (EASI) model. *Journal of Experimental Social Psychology, 46*(6), 1042–1048.

Van Kleef, G. A., Oveis, C., Van Der Löwe, I., LuoKogan, A., Goetz, J., & Keltner, D. (2008). Power, distress, and compassion: Turning a blind eye to the suffering of others. *Psychological Science, 19*(12), 1315–1322.

Vingerhoets, A. J., & Bylsma, L. M. (2016). The riddle of human emotional crying: A challenge for emotion researchers. *Emotion Review, 8*(3), 207–217.

Waber, D. P., De Moor, C., Forbes, P. W., Almli, C. R., Botteron, K. N., Leonard, G., . . . Brain Development Cooperative Group. (2007). The NIH MRI study of normal brain development: Performance of a population based sample of healthy children aged 6 to 18 years on a neuropsychological battery. *Journal of the International Neuropsychological Society, 13*(5), 729–746. doi.org/10.1017/S1355617707070841

Wechsler, D. (1955). *Manual for the Wechsler Adult Intelligence Scale.* Oxford: Psychological Corp.

Weng, H. Y., Fox, A. S., Hessenthaler, H. C., Stodola, D. E., & Davidson, R. J. (2015). The role of compassion in altruistic helping and punishment behavior. *PLoS One, 10*(12), e0143794.

Wolke, D., Copeland, W. E., Angold, A., & Costello, E. J. (2013). Impact of bullying in childhood on adult health, wealth, crime, and social outcomes. *Psychological Science, 24*(10), 1958–1970.

Woodman, T., Davis, P. A., Hardy, L., Callow, N., Glasscock, I., & Yuill-Proctor, J. (2009). Emotions and sport performance: An exploration of happiness, hope, and anger. *Journal of Sport and Exercise Psychology, 31*(2), 169–188.

World Health Organization. (2017, May 17). Cardiovascular diseases (CVDs). Retrieved from www.who.int/news-room/fact-sheets/detail/cardiovascular-diseases -(cvds)

World Health Organization. (2017, December 12). Dementia. Retrieved from www .who.int/news-room/fact-sheets/detail/dementia

World Health Organization. (2018, October 30). Diabetes. Retrieved from www .who.int/news-room/fact-sheets/detail/diabetes

World Health Organization. (2018, September 12). Cancer. Retrieved from www .who.int/news-room/fact-sheets/detail/cancer

Wright, B. L., & Loving, T. J. (2011). Health implications of conflict in close relationships. *Social and Personality Psychology Compass, 5*(8), 552–562.

Yang, H., & Yang, S. (2016). Sympathy fuels creativity: The beneficial effects of sympathy on originality. *Thinking Skills and Creativity, 21*, 132–143.

Yiend, J. (2010). The effects of emotion on attention: A review of attentional processing of emotional information. *Cognition and Emotion, 24*(1), 3–47. doi.org/10.1080 /02699930903205698

Yip, J. A., & Côté, S. (2013). The emotionally intelligent decision maker: Emotion-understanding ability reduces the effect of incidental anxiety on risk taking. *Psychological Science, 24*(1), 48–55. doi.org/10.1177/0956797612450031

Yip, J. A., Stein, D. H., Côté, S., & Carney, D. R. (2019). Follow your gut? Emotional intelligence moderates the association between physiologically measured somatic markers and risk-taking. *Emotion*. Advance online publication. doi.org/10.1037 /emo0000561

Zadra, J. R., & Clore, G. L. (2011). Emotion and perception: The role of affective information. *Wiley Interdisciplinary Reviews: Cognitive Science, 2*(6), 676–685.

Zelazo, P. D., & Müller, U. (2002). Executive function in typical and atypical development. In U. Goswami (Ed.), *Blackwell Handbook of Childhood Cognitive Development* (pp. 445–469). Hoboken, NJ: Blackwell Publishers.

Zeman, J., Cassano, M., Perry-Parrish, C., & Stegall, S. (2006). Emotion regulation in children and adolescents. *Journal of Developmental & Behavioral Pediatrics*, 27(2), 155–168. doi.org/10.1097/00004703-200604000-00014

Zimmermann, P., & Iwanski, A. (2014). Emotion regulation from early adolescence to emerging adulthood and middle adulthood: Age differences, gender differences, and emotion-specific developmental variations. *International Journal of Behavioral Development, 38(2)*, 182–194. doi.org/10.1177/0165025413515405

3. How to Become an Emotion Scientist

American Psychological Association. (2002). *The road to resilience.* Retrieved from www.apa.org/helpcenter/road-resilience

Boyce, T. W. (2019). *The Orchid and the Dandelion: Why Some Children Struggle and How All Can Thrive.* New York: Alfred A. Knopf.

Brackett, M. A., Mayer, J. D., & Warner, R. M. (2004). Emotional intelligence and its relation to everyday behaviour. *Personality and Individual Differences, 36*(6), 1387–1402. doi.org/10.1016/S0191-8869(03)00236-8

Brackett, M. A., & Rivers, S. E. (2014). Transforming students' lives with social and emotional learning. In R. Pekrun & L. Linnenbrink-Garcia (Eds.), *International Handbook of Emotions in Education* (pp. 368–388). New York: Routledge.

Brackett, M. A., Rivers, S. E., Bertoli, M. C., & Salovey, P. (2016). Emotional intelligence. In L. F. Barrett, M. Lewis, & J. M. Haviland-Jones (Eds.), *Handbook of Emotions* (pp. 513–531). New York: Guilford Publications.

Brackett, M. A., Rivers, S. E., Shiffman, S., Lerner, N., & Salovey, P. (2006). Relating emotional abilities to social functioning: A comparison of self-report and performance measures of emotional intelligence. *Journal of Personality and Social Psychology, 91*(4), 780–795. doi.org/10.1037/0022-3514.91.4.780

Brackett, M. A., & Salovey, P. (2004). Measuring emotional intelligence with the Mayer-Salovey-Caruso Emotional Intelligence Test (MSCEIT). In G. Geher (Ed.), *Measuring Emotional Intelligence: Common Ground and Controversy* (pp. 179–94). Happauge, NY: Nova Science Publishers, Inc.

Côté, S., Lopes, P. N., Salovey, P., & Miners, C. T. (2010). Emotional intelligence and leadership emergence in small groups. *Leadership Quarterly, 21*(3), 496–508. doi.org/10.1016/j.leaqua.2010.03.012

Crombie, D., Lombard, C., & Noakes, T. (2011). Increasing emotional intelligence in cricketers: An intervention study. *International Journal of Sports Science & Coaching, 6*(1), 69–86. doi.org/10.1260/1747-9541.6.1.69

Damasio, A. (2018). *The Strange Order of Things: Life, Feeling, and the Making of Cultures.* New York: Vintage Books.

Duckworth, A. (2016). *Grit: The Power of Passion and Perseverance.* New York: Scribner.

Dunn, E. W., Brackett, M. A., Ashton-James, C., Schneiderman, E., & Salovey, P. (2007). On emotionally intelligent time travel: Individual differences in affective forecasting ability. *Personality and Social Psychology Bulletin, 33*(1), 85–93. doi.org /10.1177/0146167206294201

Dweck, C. (2006). *Mindset: The New Psychology of Success.* New York: Ballantine Books.

Fernandez-Berrocal, P., Alcaide, R., Extremera, N., & Pizarro, D. (2006). The role of emotional intelligence in anxiety and depression among adolescents. *Individual Differences Research, 4*(1), 16–27. Retrieved from http://emotional.intelligence .uma.es/documentos/pdf60among_adolescents.pdf

Ivcevic, Z., & Brackett, M. (2014). Predicting school success: Comparing conscientiousness, grit, and emotion regulation ability. *Journal of Research in Personality, 52*, 29–36. doi.org/10.1016/j.jrp.2014.06.005

Ivcevic, Z., Brackett, M. A., & Mayer, J. D. (2007). Emotional intelligence and emotional creativity. *Journal of Personality, 75*(2), 199–236. doi.org/10.1111/j.1467 -6494.2007.00437.x

Kumar, S. (2014). Establishing linkages between emotional intelligence and transformational leadership. *Industrial Psychiatry Journal, 23*(1), 1–3. doi.org/10.4103 /0972-6748.144934

Martins, A., Ramalho, N., & Morin, E. (2010). A comprehensive meta-analysis of the relationship between emotional intelligence and health. *Personality and Individual Differences, 49*(6), 554–564. doi.org/10.1016/j.paid.2010.05.029

Miao, C., Humphrey, R. H., & Qian, S. (2017). A meta-analysis of emotional intelligence and work attitudes. *Journal of Occupational and Organizational Psychology, 90*(2), 177–202. doi.org/10.1111/joop.12167

Reuben, E., Sapienza, P., & Zingales, L. (2009). *Can we teach emotional intelligence.* (Unpublished manuscript.) New York: Columbia Business School, Columbia University.

Rivers, S. E., Brackett, M. A., Reyes, M. R., Mayer, J. D., Caruso, D. R., & Salovey, P. (2012). Measuring emotional intelligence in early adolescence with the MS-CEIT-YV: Psychometric properties and relationship with academic performance and psychosocial functioning. *Journal of Psychoeducational Assessment, 30*(4), 344–366. doi.org/10.1177/0734282912449443

Salovey, P., & Mayer, J. D. (1990). Emotional intelligence. *Imagination, Cognition and Personality, 9*(3), 185–211. doi.org/10.2190/DUGG-P24E-52WK-6CDG

Schutte, N. S., Malouff, J. M., Bobik, C., Coston, T. D., Greeson, C., Jedlicka, C., . . . Wendorf, G. (2001). Emotional intelligence and interpersonal relations. *Journal of Social Psychology, 141*(4), 523–536. doi.org/10.1080/00224540109600569

Sharot, T. (2011). The optimism bias. *Current Biology, 21*(23), R941–R945. doi.org/10 .1016/j.cub.2011.10.030

Tsai, J. L., Louie, J. Y., Chen, E. E., & Uchida, Y. (2007). Learning what feelings to desire: Socialization of ideal affect through children's storybooks. *Personality and Social Psychology Bulletin, 33*(1), 17–30. doi.org/10.1177/0146167206292749

Yip, J. A., & Côté, S. (2013). The emotionally intelligent decision maker: Emotion-understanding ability reduces the effect of incidental anxiety on risk taking. *Psychological Science, 24*(1), 48–55. doi.org/10.1177/0956797612450031

Zhang, H.-H., & Wang, H. (2011). A meta-analysis of the relationship between individual emotional intelligence and workplace performance. *Acta Psychologica Sinica, 43*(2), 188–202. Retrieved from http://en.cnki.com.cn/Article_en /CJFDTOTAL-XLXB201102009.htm

4. R: Recognizing Emotion

Ackerman, J. M., Shapiro, J. R., Neuberg, S. L., Kenrick, D. T., Becker, D. V., Griskevicius, V., . . . Schaller, M. (2006). They all look the same to me (unless they're angry) from out-group homogeneity to out-group heterogeneity. *Psychological Science, 17*(10), 836–840.

Adams Jr., R. B., Hess, U., & Kleck, R. E. (2015). The intersection of gender-related facial appearance and facial displays of emotion. *Emotion Review, 7*(1), 5–13.

Ambady, N., & Weisbuch, M. (2010). Nonverbal behavior. In S. T. Riske, D. T. Gilbert, & G. Lindzey (Eds.), *Handbook of Social Psychology* (vol. 5, pp. 464–497). Hoboken, NJ: John Wiley & Sons.

Aviezer, H., Hassin, R. R., Ryan, J., Grady, C., Susskind, J., Anderson, A., . . . Bentin, S. (2008). Angry, disgusted, or afraid? Studies on the malleability of emotion perception. *Psychological Science, 19*(7), 724–732.

Bar-Haim, Y., Lamy, D., Pergamin, L., Bakermans-Kranenburg, M. J., & Van Ijzendoorn, M. H. (2007). Threat-related attentional bias in anxious and nonanxious individuals: a meta-analytic study. *Psychological Bulletin, 133*(1), 1–24.

Barrett, L. F. (2017). *How Emotions Are Made: The Secret Life of the Brain.* Boston, MA: Houghton Mifflin Harcourt.

Barrett, L. F., Mesquita, B., & Gendron, M. (2011). Context in emotion perception. *Current Directions in Psychological Science, 20*(5), 286–290.

Baumeister, R. F., Bratslavsky, E., Finkenauer, C., & Vohs, K. D. (2001). Bad is stronger than good. *Review of General Psychology, 5*(4), 323–370.

Becker, M. W., & Leininger, M. (2011). Attentional selection is biased toward mood-congruent stimuli. *Emotion, 11*(5), 1248–1254.

Brackett, M. A., Patti, J., Stern, R., Rivers, S. E., Elbertson, N. A., Chisholm, C., &

Salovey, P. (2009). A sustainable, skill-based approach to building emotionally literate schools. In M. Hughes, H. L. Thompson, & J. B. Terrell (Eds.), *Handbook for Developing Emotional and Social Intelligence: Best Practices, Case Studies, and Strategies* (pp. 329–358). San Francisco, CA: Pfeiffer/John Wiley & Sons.

Brackett, M. A., & Rivers, S. E. (2014). Transforming students' lives with social and emotional learning. In R. Pekrun & L. Linnenbrink-Garcia (Eds.), *International Handbook of Emotions in Education* (pp. 368–388). New York: Routledge.

Bryant, G. A., Fessler, D. M., Fusaroli, R., Clint, E., Amir, D., Chávez, B., . . . Fux, M. (2018). The perception of spontaneous and volitional laughter across 21 societies. *Psychological Science, 29*(9), 1515–1525.

Caruso, D. R., & Salovey, P. (2004). *The Emotionally Intelligent Manager: How to Develop and Use the Four Key Emotional Skills of Leadership.* Hoboken, NJ: John Wiley & Sons.

Clark, M. S., Von Culin, K. R., Clark-Polner, E., & Lemay Jr., E. P. (2017). Accuracy and projection in perceptions of partners' recent emotional experiences: Both minds matter. *Emotion, 17*(2), 196–207.

Clore, G. L., & Huntsinger, J. R. (2007). How emotions inform judgment and regulate thought. *Trends in Cognitive Sciences, 11*(9), 393–399.

Cohen, D., & Gunz, A. (2002). As seen by the other . . . : Perspectives on the self in the memories and emotional perceptions of Easterners and Westerners. *Psychological Science, 13*(1), 55–59.

Cordaro, D. T., Keltner, D., Tshering, S., Wangchuk, D., & Flynn, L. M. (2016). The voice conveys emotion in ten globalized cultures and one remote village in Bhutan. *Emotion, 16*(1), 117–128.

Cordaro, D. T., Sun, R., Keltner, D., Kamble, S., Huddar, N., & McNeil, G. (2018). Universals and cultural variations in 22 emotional expressions across five cultures. *Emotion, 18*(1), 75–93.

Dalili, M. N., Penton-Voak, I. S., Harmer, C. J., & Munafo, M. R. (2015). Meta-analysis of emotion recognition deficits in major depressive disorder. *Psychological Medicine, 45*(6), 1135–1144.

Darwin, C., & Prodger, P. (1872/1998). *The Expression of the Emotions in Man and Animals.* Oxford: Oxford University Press.

Demenescu, L. R., Kortekaas, R., den Boer, J. A., & Aleman, A. (2010). Impaired attribution of emotion to facial expressions in anxiety and major depression. *PloS One, 5*(12), e15058.

Ekman, P. (1992). An argument for basic emotions. *Cognition & Emotion, 6*(3–4), 169–200.

Ekman, P., & Friesen, W. V. (1971). Constants across cultures in the face and emotion. *Journal of Personality and Social Psychology, 17*(2), 124–129.

Ekman, P., Friesen, W. V., & Ellsworth, P. (1972). *Emotion in the Human Face: Guidelines for Research and an Integration of Findings.* New York: Pergamon.

Elfenbein, H. A., & Ambady, N. (2003). Universals and cultural differences in recognizing emotions. *Current Directions in Psychological Science, 12*(5), 159–164.

Forgas, J. P., & Bower, G. H. (2001). Mood effects on person-perception judgments. In W. G. Parrott (Ed.), *Emotions in Social Psychology: Essential Readings* (pp. 204–215). Philadelphia: Psychology Press.

Füstös, J., Gramann, K., Herbert, B. M., & Pollatos, O. (2012). On the embodiment of emotion regulation: Interoceptive awareness facilitates reappraisal. *Social Cognitive and Affective Neuroscience, 8*(8), 911–917.

Gendron, M., Roberson, D., van der Vyver, J. M., & Barrett, L. F. (2014). Perceptions of emotion from facial expressions are not culturally universal: Evidence from a remote culture. *Emotion, 14*(2), 251–262.

Gilovich, T., Medvec, V. H., & Savitsky, K. (2000). The spotlight effect in social judgment: An egocentric bias in estimates of the salience of one's own actions and appearance. *Journal of Personality and Social Psychology, 78*(2), 211–222.

Hertenstein, M. J., Holmes, R., McCullough, M., & Keltner, D. (2009). The communication of emotion via touch. *Emotion, 9*(4), 566–573.

Hertenstein, M. J., Keltner, D., App, B., Bulleit, B. A., & Jaskolka, A. R. (2006). Touch communicates distinct emotions. *Emotion, 6*(3), 528–533.

Hess, U., Adams Jr, R. B., & Kleck, R. E. (2004). Facial appearance, gender, and emotion expression. *Emotion, 4*(4), 378–388.

Hess, U., Adams, R. B., Grammer, K., & Kleck, R. E. (2009). Face gender and emotion expression: Are angry women more like men? *Journal of Vision, 9*(12), article 19.

Isbell, L. M., & Lair, E. C. (2013). Moods, emotions, and evaluations as information. In D. Carlston (Ed.), *The Oxford Handbook of Social Cognition* (pp. 435–462). New York: Oxford University Press.

Ito, T., Yokokawa, K., Yahata, N., Isato, A., Suhara, T., & Yamada, M. (2017). Neural basis of negativity bias in the perception of ambiguous facial expression. *Scientific Reports, 7*(1), 420.

Izard, C. E., Woodburn, E. M., Finlon, K. J., Krauthamer-Ewing, E. S., Grossman, S. R., & Seidenfeld, A. (2011). Emotion knowledge, emotion utilization, and emotion regulation. *Emotion Review, 3*(1), 44–52.

Joseph, D. L., & Newman, D. A. (2010). Emotional intelligence: An integrative meta-analysis and cascading model. *Journal of Applied Psychology, 95*(1), 54–78.

Knapp, M. L., Hall, J. A., & Horgan, T. G. (2013). *Nonverbal Communication in Human Interaction.* Boston, MA: Cengage Learning.

Knyazev, G. G., Bocharov, A. V., Slobodskaya, H. R., & Ryabichenko, T. I. (2008).

Personality-linked biases in perception of emotional facial expressions. *Personality and Individual Differences, 44*(5), 1093–1104.

Krumhuber, E., & Kappas, A. (2005). Moving smiles: The role of dynamic components for the perception of the genuineness of smiles. *Journal of Nonverbal Behavior, 29*(1), 3–24.

Lewis, M. D. (2005). Bridging emotion theory and neurobiology through dynamic systems modeling. *Behavioral and Brain Sciences, 28*(2), 169–194.

Matsumoto, D. (1999). American-Japanese cultural differences in judgements of expression intensity and subjective experience. *Cognition & Emotion, 13*(2), 201–218.

Matsumoto, D., & Ekman, P. (1989). American-Japanese cultural differences in intensity ratings of facial expressions of emotion. *Motivation and Emotion, 13*(2), 143–157.

Mesquita, B., De Leersnyder, J., & Boiger, M. (2016). The cultural psychology of emotions. In L. F. Barrett, M. Lewis, & J. M. Haviland-Jones (Eds.), *Handbook of Emotions* (pp. 393–-411). New York: Guilford Publications.

Nathanson, L., Rivers, S. E., Flynn, L. M., & Brackett, M. A. (2016). Creating emotionally intelligent schools with RULER. *Emotion Review, 8*(4), 305–310.

Pope, A. (1903). *Essay on criticism.* London: JM Dent.

Roseman, I. J. (2013). Appraisal in the emotion system: Coherence in strategies for coping. *Emotion Review, 5*(2), 141–149.

Rosenthal, R. (2003). Covert communication in laboratories, classrooms, and the truly real world. *Current Directions in Psychological Science, 12*(5), 151–154.

Rozin, P., & Royzman, E. B. (2001). Negativity bias, negativity dominance, and contagion. *Personality and Social Psychology Review, 5*(4), 296–320.

Russell, J. A. (1980). A circumplex model of affect. *Journal of Personality and Social Psychology, 39*(6), 1161–1178.

Schönenberg, M., & Jusyte, A. (2014). Investigation of the hostile attribution bias toward ambiguous facial cues in antisocial violent offenders. *European Archives of Psychiatry and Clinical Neuroscience, 264*(1), 61–69.

Wang, Q., Chen, G., Wang, Z., Hu, C. S., Hu, X., & Fu, G. (2014). Implicit racial attitudes influence perceived emotional intensity on other-race faces. *PloS One, 9*(8), e105946.

Weiss, B., Dodge, K. A., Bates, J. E., & Pettit, G. S. (1992). Some consequences of early harsh discipline: Child aggression and a maladaptive social information processing style. *Child Development, 63*(6), 1321–1335.

Widmeyer, W. N., & Loy, J. W. (1988). When you're hot, you're hot! Warm-cold effects in first impressions of persons and teaching effectiveness. *Journal of Educational Psychology, 80*(1), 118–121.

5. U: Understanding Emotion

Bowers, M. E., & Yehuda, R. (2016). Intergenerational transmission of stress in humans. *Neuropsychopharmacology, 41*(1), 232–244.

Brackett, M. A., Patti, J., Stern, R., Rivers, S. E., Elbertson, N. A., Chisholm, C., & Salovey, P. (2009). A sustainable, skill-based approach to building emotionally literate schools. In M. Hughes, H. L. Thompson, & J. B. Terrell (Eds.), *Handbook for Developing Emotional and Social Intelligence: Best Practices, Case Studies, and Strategies* (pp. 329–358). San Francisco, CA: Pfeiffer/John Wiley & Sons.

Brackett, M. A., & Rivers, S. E. (2014). Transforming students' lives with social and emotional learning. In R. Pekrun & L. Linnenbrink-Garcia (Eds.), *International Handbook of Emotions in Education* (pp. 368–388). New York: Routledge.

Campos, B., Shiota, M. N., Keltner, D., Gonzaga, G. C., & Goetz, J. L. (2013). What is shared, what is different? Core relational themes and expressive displays of eight positive emotions. *Cognition & Emotion, 27*(1), 37–52.

Clore, G. L. & Schiller, A. J. (2016). New light on the affect-cognition connection. In L. F. Barrett, M. Lewis, & J. M. Haviland-Jones (Eds.), *Handbook of Emotions* (pp. 532–546). New York: Guilford Publications.

Cordaro, D. T., Brackett, M., Glass, L., & Anderson, C. L. (2016). Contentment: Perceived completeness across cultures and traditions. *Review of General Psychology, 20*(3), 221–235.

Dekel, R., & Goldblatt, H. (2008). Is there intergenerational transmission of trauma? The case of combat veterans' children. *American Journal of Orthopsychiatry, 78*(3), 281–289.

Fredrickson, B. L. (2013). Positive emotions broaden and build. In P. Devine & A. Plant (Eds.), *Advances in Experimental Social Psychology* (vol. 47, pp. 1–53). Cambridge, MA: Academic Press.

Genzel, B., Rarick, J. R. D., & Morris, P. A. (2016). Stress and emotion: Embodied, in context, and across the lifespan. In L. F. Barrett, M. Lewis, & J. M. Haviland-Jones (Eds.), *Handbook of Emotions* (pp. 707–735). New York: Guilford Publications.

Kelley, H. H., & Michela, J. L. (1980). Attribution theory and research. *Annual Review of Psychology, 31*(1), 457–501.

Lazarus, R. S. (1991). Progress on a cognitive-motivational-relational theory of emotion. *American Psychologist, 46*(8), 819–834.

Lewis, M. (2016). Self-conscious emotions: Embarrassment, pride, shame, guilt, and hubris. In L. F. Barrett, M. Lewis, & J. M. Haviland-Jones (Eds.), *Handbook of Emotions* (pp. 792–814). New York: Guilford Publications.

Lupien, S. J., McEwen, B. S., Gunnar, M. R., & Heim, C. (2009). Effects of stress throughout the lifespan on the brain, behaviour and cognition. *Nature Reviews Neuroscience, 10*, 434–445.

Mendes, W. B. (2016). Emotion and the autonomic nervous system. In L. F. Barrett, M. Lewis, & J. M. Haviland-Jones (Eds.), *Handbook of Emotions* (pp. 166–181). New York: Guilford Publications.

Moeller, J., Ivcevic, Z., Brackett, M. A., & White, A. E. (2018). Mixed emotions: Network analyses of intra-individual co-occurrences within and across situations. *Emotion, 18*(8), 1106–1121.

Moors, A., Ellsworth, P. C., Scherer, K. R., & Frijda, N. H. (2013). Appraisal theories of emotion: State of the art and future development. *Emotion Review, 5*(2), 119–124.

Nathanson, L., Rivers, S. E., Flynn, L. M., & Brackett, M. A. (2016). Creating emotionally intelligent schools with RULER. *Emotion Review, 8*(4), 305–310.

Parrott, W. G., & Smith, R. H. (1993). Distinguishing the experiences of envy and jealousy. *Journal of Personality and Social Psychology, 64*(6), 906–920.

Roseman, I. J. (1991). Appraisal determinants of discrete emotions. *Cognition & Emotion, 5*(3), 161–200.

Roseman, I. J. (2013). Appraisal in the emotion system: Coherence in strategies for coping. *Emotion Review, 5*(2), 141–149.

Russell, J. A. (1980). A circumplex model of affect. *Journal of Personality and Social Psychology, 39*(6), 1161–1178.

Salovey, P. (Ed.). (1991). *The Psychology of Jealousy and Envy.* New York: Guilford Press.

Scherer, K. R., Schorr, A., & Johnstone, T. (Eds.). (2001). *Appraisal Processes in Emotion: Theory, Methods, Research.* New York: Oxford University Press.

Shields, G. S., Sazma, M. A., & Yonelinas, A. P. (2016). The effects of acute stress on core executive functions: A meta-analysis and comparison with cortisol. *Neuroscience & Biobehavioral Reviews, 68*, 651–668.

Steinberg, L. (2005). Cognitive and affective development in adolescence. *Trends in Cognitive Sciences, 9*(2), 69–74.

Tracy, J. L., & Robins, R. W. (2006). Appraisal antecedents of shame and guilt: Support for a theoretical model. *Personality and Social Psychology Bulletin, 32*(10), 1339–1351.

Weiner, B. (1985). An attributional theory of achievement motivation and emotion. *Psychological Review, 92*(4), 548–573.

Weisinger, H., & Pawliw-Fry, J. P. (2015). *Performing Under Pressure: The Science of Doing Your Best When it Matters Most.* New York: Crown Publishing.

Zeman, J., Cassano, M., Perry-Parrish, C., & Stegall, S. (2006). Emotion regulation in children and adolescents. *Journal of Developmental & Behavioral Pediatrics, 27*(2), 155–168.

Zimmermann, P., & Iwanski, A. (2014). Emotion regulation from early adolescence to emerging adulthood and middle adulthood: Age differences, gender differences, and emotion-specific developmental variations. *International Journal of Behavioral Development, 38*(2), 182–194.

6. L: Labeling Emotion

Barrett, L. F. (2006). Solving the emotion paradox: Categorization and the experience of emotion. *Personality and Social Psychology Review, 10*(1), 20–46.

Barrett, L. F. (2017). *How Emotions Are Made: The Secret Life of the Brain*. Boston: Houghton Mifflin Harcourt.

Barrett, L. F. (2017). The theory of constructed emotion: An active inference account of interoception and categorization. *Social Cognitive and Affective Neuroscience, 12*(1), 1–23.

Barrett, L. F., Gross, J., Christensen, T. C., & Benvenuto, M. (2001). Knowing what you're feeling and knowing what to do about it: Mapping the relation between emotion differentiation and emotion regulation. *Cognition and Emotion, 15*(6), 713–724.

Baumeister, R. F., Bratslavsky, E., Finkenauer, C., & Vohs, K. D. (2001). Bad is stronger than good. *Review of General Psychology, 5*(4), 323–370.

Bird, G., & Cook, R. (2013). Mixed emotions: The contribution of alexithymia to the emotional symptoms of autism. *Translational Psychiatry, 3*(7), e285.

Camras, L. A., Fatani, S. S., Fraumeni, B. R., & Shuster, M. M. (2016). The development of facial expressions: Current perspectives on infant emotions. In L. F. Barrett, M. Lewis, & J. M. Haviland-Jones (Eds.), *Handbook of Emotions* (pp. 255–271). New York: Guilford Publications.

Cosmides, L., & Tooby, J. (2000). Evolutionary psychology and the emotions. In M. Lewis & J. M. Haviland-Jones (Eds.), *Handbook of Emotions* (pp. 91–115). New York: Guilford Publications.

Creswell, J. D., Way, B. M., Eisenberger, N. I., & Lieberman, M. D. (2007). Neural correlates of dispositional mindfulness during affect labeling. *Psychosomatic Medicine, 69*(6), 560–565.

Demaree, H. A., Everhart, D. E., Youngstrom, E. A., & Harrison, D. W. (2005). Brain lateralization of emotional processing: Historical roots and a future incorporating "dominance." *Behavioral and Cognitive Neuroscience Reviews, 4*(1), 3–20.

Durkin, K., & Conti-Ramsden, G. (2010). Young people with specific language impairment: A review of social and emotional functioning in adolescence. *Child Language Teaching and Therapy, 26*(2), 105–121.

Durlak, J. A., Weissberg, R. P., Dymnicki, A. B., Taylor, R. D., & Schellinger, K. B. (2011). The impact of enhancing students' social and emotional learning: A meta-analysis of school-based universal interventions. *Child Development, 82*(1), 405–432.

Eisenberg, N., Sadovsky, A., & Spinrad, T. L. (2005). Associations of emotion-related regulation with language skills, emotion knowledge, and academic outcomes. *New Directions for Child and Adolescent Development, 2005*(109), 109–118.

Elert, E. (2013, January 4). 21 emotions for which there are no English words [infographic]. *Popular Science*. Retrieved from www.popsci.com/science/article/2013 -01/emotions-which-there-are-no-english-words-infographic

Harris, P. L., de Rosnay, M., & Pons, F. (2016). Understanding emotion. In L. F. Barrett, M. Lewis, & J. M. Haviland-Jones (Eds.), *Handbook of Emotions* (pp. 293–306). New York: Guilford Publications.

Hart, B., & Risley, T. R. (1995). *Meaningful Differences in the Everyday Experience of Young American Children*. Baltimore, MD: Paul H. Brookes Publishing.

Hussein, B. A. S. (2012). The Sapir-Whorf hypothesis today. *Theory and Practice in Language Studies, 2*(3), 642–646.

Izard, C. E., Woodburn, E. M., Finlon, K. J., Krauthamer-Ewing, E. S., Grossman, S. R., & Seidenfeld, A. (2011). Emotion knowledge, emotion utilization, and emotion regulation. *Emotion Review, 3*(1), 44–52.

Izard, C., Fine, S., Schultz, D., Mostow, A., Ackerman, B., & Youngstrom, E. (2001). Emotion knowledge as a predictor of social behavior and academic competence in children at risk. *Psychological Science, 12*(1), 18–23.

Kashdan, T. B., Barrett, L. F., & McKnight, P. E. (2015). Unpacking emotion differentiation: Transforming unpleasant experience by perceiving distinctions in negativity. *Current Directions in Psychological Science, 24*(1), 10–16.

Kircanski, K., Lieberman, M. D., & Craske, M. G. (2012). Feelings into words: Contributions of language to exposure therapy. *Psychological Science, 23*(10), 1086–1091.

Larsen, J. K., Brand, N., Bermond, B., & Hijman, R. (2003). Cognitive and emotional characteristics of alexithymia: A review of neurobiological studies. *Journal of Psychosomatic Research, 54*(6), 533–541.

Lewis, M. (2016). The emergence of human emotions. In L. F. Barrett, M. Lewis, & J. M. Haviland-Jones (Eds.), *Handbook of Emotions* (pp. 272–292). New York: Guilford Publications.

Li, J., Wang, L., & Fischer, K. (2004). The organisation of Chinese shame concepts? *Cognition and Emotion, 18*(6), 767–797.

Lieberman, M. D., Eisenberger, N. I., Crockett, M. J., Tom, S. M., Pfeifer, J. H., & Way, B. M. (2007). Putting feelings into words. *Psychological Science, 18*(5), 421–428.

Lieberman, M. D., Inagaki, T. K., Tabibnia, G., & Crockett, M. J. (2011). Subjective responses to emotional stimuli during labeling, reappraisal, and distraction. *Emotion, 11*(3), 468–480.

Lindquist, K. A., Gendron, M., & Satpute, A. B. (2016). Language and emotion: Putting words into feelings and feelings into words. In L. F. Barrett, M. Lewis, & J. M. Haviland-Jones (Eds.), *Handbook of Emotions* (pp. 579–594). New York: Guilford Publications.

Mohammad, S. M., & Turney, P. D. (2010, June). Emotions evoked by common words and phrases: Using mechanical turk to create an emotion lexicon. In Proceedings of the NAACL HLT 2010 workshop on computational approaches to analysis and generation of emotion in text (pp. 26–34). Stroudsburg, PA: Association for Computational Linguistics.

Pennebaker, J. W. (1993). Putting stress into words: Health, linguistic, and therapeutic implications. *Behaviour Research and Therapy, 31*(6), 539–548.

Pennebaker, J. W. (2018). Expressive writing in psychological science. *Perspectives on Psychological Science, 13*(2), 226–229.

Robson, D. (2017, January 26). The "untranslatable" emotions you never knew you had. BBC. Retrieved from www.bbc.com/future/story/20170126-the-untranslatable-emotions-you-never-knew-you-had

Rozin, P., & Royzman, E. B. (2001). Negativity bias, negativity dominance, and contagion. *Personality and Social Psychology Review, 5*(4), 296–320.

Schrauf, R. W., & Sanchez, J. (2004). The preponderance of negative emotion words in the emotion lexicon: A cross-generational and cross-linguistic study. *Journal of Multilingual and Multicultural Development, 25*(2–3), 266–284.

Sperry, D. E., Sperry, L. L., & Miller, P. J. (in press). Reexamining the verbal environments of children from different Socioeconomic backgrounds. *Child Development.*

St. Clair, M. C., Pickles, A., Durkin, K., & Conti-Ramsden, G. (2011). A longitudinal study of behavioral, emotional and social difficulties in individuals with a history of specific language impairment (SLI). *Journal of Communication Disorders, 44*(2), 186–199.

Taylor, G. J., & Bagby, R. M. (2000). An overview of the alexithymia construct. In R. Bar-On & J. D. A. Parker (Eds.), *The Handbook of Emotional Intelligence: Theory, Development, Assessment, and Application at Home, School, and in the Workplace* (pp. 40–67). San Francisco, CA: Jossey-Bass.

Toivonen, R., Kivelä, M., Saramäki, J., Viinikainen, M., Vanhatalo, M., & Sams, M. (2012). Networks of emotion concepts. *PLoS One, 7*(1), e28883.

Torre, J. B., & Lieberman, M. D. (2018). Putting feelings into words: Affect labeling as implicit emotion regulation. *Emotion Review, 10*(2), 116–124.

Torrisi, S. J., Lieberman, M. D., Bookheimer, S. Y., & Altshuler, L. L. (2013).

Advancing understanding of affect labeling with dynamic causal modeling. *NeuroImage, 82*, 481–488.

Tugade, M. M., Fredrickson, B. L., & Feldman Barrett, L. (2004). Psychological resilience and positive emotional granularity: Examining the benefits of positive emotions on coping and health. *Journal of Personality, 72*(6), 1161–1190.

Weisleder, A., & Fernald, A. (2013). Talking to children matters: Early language experience strengthens processing and builds vocabulary. *Psychological Science, 24*(11), 2143–2152.

Widen, S. C. (2016). The development of children's concepts of emotion. In L. F. Barrett, M. Lewis, & J. M. Haviland-Jones (Eds.), *Handbook of Emotions* (pp. 307–318). New York: Guilford Publications.

Wierzbicka, A. (2006). *English: Meaning and Culture.* New York: Oxford University Press.

Yew, S. G. K., & O'Kearney, R. (2013). Emotional and behavioural outcomes later in childhood and adolescence for children with specific language impairments: Meta-analyses of controlled prospective studies. *Journal of Child Psychology and Psychiatry, 54*(5), 516–524.

7. E: Expressing Emotion

Barrett, L. F. (2017). *How Emotions Are Made: The Secret Life of the Brain.* Boston: Houghton Mifflin Harcourt.

Barrett, L. F., Lewis, M., & Haviland-Jones, J. M. (Eds.). (2016). *Handbook of Emotions.* New York: Guilford Publications.

Brody, L. R. (1993). On understanding gender differences in the expression of emotion. In S. L. Ablon, D. P. Brown, E. J. Khantzian, & J. E. Mack (Eds.), *Human Feelings: Explorations in Affect Development and Meaning* (pp. 87–121). Hillsdale, NJ: Analytic Press, Inc.

Brody, L. R. (2000). The socialization of gender differences in emotional expression: Display rules, infant temperament, and differentiation. *Gender and Emotion: Social Psychological Perspectives, 2*, 24–47. doi.org/10.1017/CBO9780511628191.003

Buck, R. (1977). Nonverbal communication of affect in preschool children: Relationships with personality and skin conductance. *Journal of Personality and Social Psychology, 35*(4), 225–236.

Buck, R. (1984). *The Communication of Emotion.* New York: Guilford Press.

Chaplin, T. M., & Aldao, A. (2013). Gender differences in emotion expression in children: A meta-analytic review. *Psychological Bulletin, 139*(4), 735–765.

Chaplin, T. M., Hong, K., Bergquist, K., & Sinha, R. (2008). Gender differences in response to emotional stress: an assessment across subjective, behavioral, and physiological domains and relations to alcohol craving. *Alcoholism: Clinical and Experimental Research, 32*(7), 1242–1250.

Danner, D. D., Snowdon, D. A., & Friesen, W. V. (2001). Positive emotions in early life and longevity: Findings from the nun study. *Journal of Personality and Social Psychology, 80*(5), 804–813.

Darwin, C., & Prodger, P. (1998). *The Expression of the Emotions in Man and Animals.* Oxford: Oxford University Press.

Domagalski, T. A., & Steelman, L. A. (2007). The impact of gender and organizational status on workplace anger expression. *Management Communication Quarterly, 20*(3), 297–315.

Ekman, P. (2009). Lie catching and microexpressions. In C. Martin (Ed.), *The Philosophy of Deception* (pp. 118–137). Oxford: Oxford University Press.

Finkenauer, C., & Rimé, B. (1998). Keeping emotional memories secret: Health and subjective well-being when emotions are not shared. *Journal of Health Psychology, 3*(1), 47–58.

Friesen, W. V. (1972). *Cultural differences in facial expressions in a social situation: An experimental test of the concept of display rules* (Unpublished doctoral dissertation). University of California–San Francisco, San Francisco, CA.

Grandey, A. A. (2015). Smiling for a wage: What emotional labor teaches us about emotion regulation. *Psychological Inquiry, 26*(1), 54–60.

Grandey, A., Foo, S. C., Groth, M., & Goodwin, R. E. (2012). Free to be you and me: A climate of authenticity alleviates burnout from emotional labor. *Journal of Occupational Health Psychology, 17*(1), 1–14.

Gross, J. J., & John, O. P. (1997). Revealing feelings: Facets of emotional expressivity in self-reports, peer ratings, and behavior. *Journal of Personality and Social Psychology, 72*(2), 435–448.

Hagenauer, G., & Volet, S. E. (2014). "I don't hide my feelings, even though I try to": Insight into teacher educator emotion display. *Australian Educational Researcher, 41*(3), 261–281.

Hall, J. A., Carter, J. D., & Horgan, T. G. (2000). Gender differences in nonverbal communication of emotion. In A. H. Fischer (Ed.), *Studies in Emotion and Social Interaction. Second series. Gender and Emotion: Social Psychological Perspectives* (pp. 97–117). New York: Cambridge University Press. doi.org/10.1017/CBO9780511628191.006

Hall, J. A., & Schmid Mast, M. (2008). Are women always more interpersonally sensitive than men? Impact of goals and content domain. *Personality and Social Psychology Bulletin, 34*(1), 144–155.

Harker, L., & Keltner, D. (2001). Expressions of positive emotion in women's college yearbook pictures and their relationship to personality and life outcomes across adulthood. *Journal of Personality and Social Psychology, 80*(1), 112–124.

Hertenstein, M. J., Hansel, C. A., Butts, A. M., & Hile, S. N. (2009). Smile intensity in photographs predicts divorce later in life. *Motivation and Emotion, 33*(2), 99–105.

Hochschild, A. R. (2012). *The Managed Heart: Commercialization of Human Feeling.* Oakland, CA: University of California Press.

Johnston, V. S. (1999). *Why We Feel: The Science of Human Emotions.* New York: Perseus Publishing.

Kirschbaum, C., Kudielka, B. M., Gaab, J., Schommer, N. C., & Hellhammer, D. H. (1999). Impact of gender, menstrual cycle phase, and oral contraceptives on the activity of the hypothalamus-pituitary-adrenal axis. *Psychosomatic Medicine, 61*(2), 154–162.

Kotchemidova, C. (2005). From good cheer to "drive-by smiling": A social history of cheerfulness. *Journal of Social History, 39*(1), 5–37.

Kring, A. M., & Gordon, A. H. (1998). Sex differences in emotion: Expression, experience, and physiology. *Journal of Personality and Social Psychology, 74*(3), 686–703.

LaFrance, M., Hecht, M. A., & Paluck, E. L. (2003). The contingent smile: A meta-analysis of sex differences in smiling. *Psychological Bulletin, 129*(2), 305–334.

Lease, S. H. (2018). Assertive behavior: A double-edged sword for women at work? *Clinical Psychology: Science and Practice, 25*(1), e12226.

Leitenberg, H., Greenwald, E., & Cado, S. (1992). A retrospective study of long-term methods of coping with having been sexually abused during childhood. *Child Abuse & Neglect, 16*(3), 399–407.

Levenson, R. W., Carstensen, L. L., & Gottman, J. M. (1994). Influence of age and gender on affect, physiology, and their interrelations: A study of long-term marriages. *Journal of Personality and Social Psychology, 67*(1), 56–68.

Machiavelli, N. (2008). *The Prince.* Indianapolis, IL: Hackett Publishing.

Matsumoto, D. (1990). Cultural similarities and differences in display rules. *Motivation and Emotion, 14*(3), 195–214.

Nelson, J. A., Leerkes, E. M., O'Brien, M., Calkins, S. D., & Marcovitch, S. (2012). African American and European American mothers' beliefs about negative emotions and emotion socialization practices. *Parenting, 12*(1), 22–41.

Oatley, K., Keltner, D., & Jenkins, J. M. (2006). *Understanding Emotions.* Hoboken, NJ: Blackwell Publishing.

Pennebaker, J. W. (1995). *Emotion, Disclosure, & Health.* Washington, DC: American Psychological Association.

Pennebaker, J. W. (1997). Writing about emotional experiences as a therapeutic process. *Psychological Science, 8*(3), 162–166.

Pennebaker, J. W., Kiecolt-Glaser, J. K., & Glaser, R. (1988). Disclosure of traumas and immune function: Health implications for psychotherapy. *Journal of Consulting and Clinical Psychology, 56*(2), 239–245.

Randolph, S. M., Koblinsky, S. A., & Roberts, D. D. (1996). Studying the role of family and school in the development of African American preschoolers in violent neighborhoods. *Journal of Negro Education,* 282–294.

Roorda, D. L., Koomen, H. M., Spilt, J. L., & Oort, F. J. (2011). The influence of affective teacher–student relationships on students' school engagement and achievement: A meta-analytic approach. *Review of Educational Research, 81*(4), 493–529.

Sheldon, K. M., Titova, L., Gordeeva, T. O., Osin, E. N., Lyubomirsky, S., & Bogomaz, S. (2017). Russians inhibit the expression of happiness to strangers: Testing a display rule model. *Journal of Cross-Cultural Psychology, 48*(5), 718–733.

Tracy, J. L., & Matsumoto, D. (2008). The spontaneous expression of pride and shame: Evidence for biologically innate nonverbal displays. *Proceedings of the National Academy of Sciences, 105*(33), 11655–11660.

Tronick, E. Z. (1989). Emotions and emotional communication in infants. *American Psychologist, 44*(2), 112–119.

Tsai, J. L., Ang, J. Y. Z., Blevins, E., Goernandt, J., Fung, H. H., Jiang, D., . . . Haddouk, L. (2016). Leaders' smiles reflect cultural differences in ideal affect. *Emotion, 16*(2), 183–195.

Uono, S., & Hietanen, J. K. (2015). Eye contact perception in the West and East: A cross-cultural study. *Plos One, 10*(2), e0118094.

Waldstein, D. (2018, September 8). Serena Williams accuses official of sexism in U.S. Open loss to Naomi Osaka. *New York Times.* Retrieved from www.nytimes.com /2018/09/08/sports/serena-williams-vs-naomi-osaka-us-open.html

Wallbott, H. G. (1998). Bodily expression of emotion. *European Journal of Social Psychology, 28*(6), 879–896.

Walsh, K., Fortier, M. A., & DiLillo, D. (2010). Adult coping with childhood sexual abuse: A theoretical and empirical review. *Aggression and Violent Behavior, 15*(1), 1–13.

8. R: Regulating Emotion

Alderman, L. (2016, November 9). Breathe. Exhale. Repeat: The benefits of controlled breathing. *New York Times.* Retrieved from www.nytimes.com/2016 /11/09/well/mind/breathe-exhale-repeat-the-benefits-of-controlled-breathing .html

Alvaro, P. K., Roberts, R. M., & Harris, J. K. (2013). A systematic review assessing bidirectionality between sleep disturbances, anxiety, and depression. *Sleep, 36*(7), 1059–1068.

Astin, J. A. (1997). Stress reduction through mindfulness meditation. *Psychotherapy and Psychosomatics, 66*(2), 97–106.

Bariola, E., Gullone, E., & Hughes, E. K. (2011). Child and adolescent emotion regulation: The role of parental emotion regulation and expression. *Clinical Child and Family Psychology Review, 14*(2), 198.

Bariso, J. (2018, February 28). 13 signs of high emotional intelligence. *Inc.* Retrieved from www.inc.com/justin-bariso/13-things-emotionally-intelligent-people-do .html

Barrett, L. F., Gross, J., Christensen, T. C., & Benvenuto, M. (2001). Knowing what you're feeling and knowing what to do about it: Mapping the relation between emotion differentiation and emotion regulation. *Cognition & Emotion, 15*(6), 713–724.

Beilharz, J., Maniam, J., & Morris, M. (2015). Diet-induced cognitive deficits: The role of fat and sugar, potential mechanisms and nutritional interventions. *Nutrients, 7*(8), 6719–6738.

Black, D. S., & Slavich, G. M. (2016). Mindfulness meditation and the immune system: A systematic review of randomized controlled trials. *Annals of the New York Academy of Sciences, 1373*(1), 13–24.

Brooks, A. W. (2014). Get excited: Reappraising pre-performance anxiety as excitement. *Journal of Experimental Psychology: General, 143*(3), 1144–1158.

Brown, K. W., & Ryan, R. M. (2003). The benefits of being present: Mindfulness and its role in psychological well-being. *Journal of Personality and Social Psychology, 84*(4), 822–848.

Burg, J. M., & Michalak, J. (2011). The healthy quality of mindful breathing: Associations with rumination and depression. *Cognitive Therapy and Research, 35*(2), 179–185.

Butler, E. A., & Randall, A. K. (2013). Emotional coregulation in close relationships. *Emotion Review, 5*(2), 202–210.

Cho, H., Ryu, S., Noh, J., & Lee, J. (2016). The effectiveness of daily mindful breathing practices on test anxiety of students. *PloS One, 11*(10), e0164822.

Cohen, S. (2004). Social relationships and health. *American Psychologist, 59*(8), 676.

Consolo, K., Fusner, S., & Staib, S. (2008). Effects of diaphragmatic breathing on stress levels of nursing students. *Teaching and Learning in Nursing, 3*(2), 67–71.

Crum, A. (2011). Evaluating a mindset training program to unleash the enhancing nature of stress. In *Academy of Management Proceedings* (vol. 2011, no. 1, pp. 1–6). Briarcliff Manor, NY: Academy of Management.

Crum, A. J., Akinola, M., Martin, A., & Fath, S. (2017). The role of stress mindset in shaping cognitive, emotional, and physiological responses to challenging and threatening stress. *Anxiety, Stress, & Coping, 30*(4), 379–395.

Crum, A., & Lyddy, C. (2014). De-stressing stress: The power of mindsets and the art of stressing mindfully. In A. Ie, C. Ngnoumen, & E. J. Langer (Eds.), *The Wiley Blackwell Handbook of Mindfulness* (vol. 1, pp. 948–963). Malden, MA: John Wiley & Sons.

Crum, A. J., Salovey, P., & Achor, S. (2013). Rethinking stress: The role of mindsets in determining the stress response. *Journal of Personality and Social Psychology, 104*(4), 716–733.

Deslandes, A., Moraes, H., Ferreira, C., Veiga, H., Silveira, H., Mouta, R., . . . Laks, J. (2009). Exercise and mental health: Many reasons to move. *Neuropsychobiology, 59*(4), 191–198.

Dobson, K. S., & Dozois, D. J. (Eds.). (2019). *Handbook of Cognitive-Behavioral Therapies.* New York: Guilford Publications.

Drabant, E. M., McRae, K., Manuck, S. B., Hariri, A. R., & Gross, J. J. (2009). Individual differences in typical reappraisal use predict amygdala and prefrontal responses. *Biological Psychiatry, 65*(5), 367–373.

Evans, C. A., & Porter, C. L. (2009). The emergence of mother–infant co-regulation during the first year: Links to infants' developmental status and attachment. *Infant Behavior and Development, 32*(2), 147–158.

Feldman, G., Greeson, J., & Senville, J. (2010). Differential effects of mindful breathing, progressive muscle relaxation, and loving-kindness meditation on decentering and negative reactions to repetitive thoughts. *Behaviour Research and Therapy, 48*(10), 1002–1011.

Gross, J. J. (1998). Antecedent- and response-focused emotion regulation: Divergent consequences for experience, expression, and physiology. *Journal of Personality and Social Psychology, 74*(1), 224–237.

Gross, J. J. (1998). The emerging field of emotion regulation: An integrative review. *Review of General Psychology, 2*(3), 271–299.

Gross, J. J. (2001). Emotion regulation in adulthood: Timing is everything. *Current Directions in Psychological Science, 10*(6), 214–219.

Grossman, P., Niemann, L., Schmidt, S., & Walach, H. (2004). Mindfulness-based stress reduction and health benefits: A meta-analysis. *Journal of Psychosomatic Research, 57*(1), 35–43.

Herrero, J. L., Khuvis, S., Yeagle, E., Cerf, M., & Mehta, A. D. (2017). Breathing above the brainstem: Volitional control and attentional modulation in humans. *Journal of Neurophysiology, 119*(1), 145–159.

Hofmann, S. G., Heering, S., Sawyer, A. T., & Asnaani, A. (2009). How to handle anxiety: The effects of reappraisal, acceptance, and suppression strategies on anxious arousal. *Behaviour Research and Therapy, 47*(5), 389–394.

Hülsheger, U. R., Alberts, H. J., Feinholdt, A., & Lang, J. W. (2013). Benefits of mindfulness at work: The role of mindfulness in emotion regulation, emotional exhaustion, and job satisfaction. *Journal of Applied Psychology, 98*(2), 310–325.

Jamieson, J. P., Crum, A. J., Goyer, J. P., Marotta, M. E., & Akinola, M. (2018). Optimizing stress responses with reappraisal and mindset interventions: An integrated model. *Anxiety, Stress, & Coping, 31*(3), 245–261.

Jamieson, J. P., Mendes, W. B., Blackstock, E., & Schmader, T. (2010). Turning the knots in your stomach into bows: Reappraising arousal improves performance on the GRE. *Journal of Experimental Social Psychology, 46*(1), 208–212.

Johnson, D. R. (2009). Emotional attention set-shifting and its relationship to anxiety and emotion regulation. *Emotion, 9*(5), 681–690.

Kingston, J., Chadwick, P., Meron, D., & Skinner, T. C. (2007). A pilot randomized control trial investigating the effect of mindfulness practice on pain tolerance, psychological well-being, and physiological activity. *Journal of Psychosomatic Research, 62*(3), 297–300.

Kross, E., & Ayduk, O. (2017). Self-distancing: Theory, research, and current directions. In J. Olsen (Ed.), *Advances in Experimental Social Psychology* (vol. 55, pp. 81–136). Cambridge, MA: Academic Press.

Kross, E., Bruehlman-Senecal, E., Park, J., Burson, A., Dougherty, A., Shablack, H., . . . Ayduk, O. (2014). Self-talk as a regulatory mechanism: How you do it matters. *Journal of Personality and Social Psychology, 106*(2), 304–324.

LeDoux, J. (1998). *The Emotional Brain: The Mysterious Underpinnings of Emotional Life.* New York: Simon & Schuster.

Levenson, R. W. (2014). The autonomic nervous system and emotion. *Emotion Review, 6*(2), 100–112.

Ma, X., Yue, Z. Q., Gong, Z. Q., Zhang, H., Duan, N. Y., Shi, Y. T., . . . Li, Y. F. (2017). The effect of diaphragmatic breathing on attention, negative affect and stress in healthy adults. *Frontiers in Psychology, 8*, 874.

Mangelsdorf, S. C., Shapiro, J. R., & Marzolf, D. (1995). Developmental and temperamental differences in emotion regulation in infancy. *Child Development, 66*(6), 1817–1828.

Mauss, I. B., Troy, A. S., & LeBourgeois, M. K. (2013). Poorer sleep quality is associated with lower emotion-regulation ability in a laboratory paradigm. *Cognition & Emotion, 27*(3), 567–576.

McRae, K., Ciesielski, B., & Gross, J. J. (2012). Unpacking cognitive reappraisal: Goals, tactics, and outcomes. *Emotion, 12*(2), 250–255.

McRae, K., Jacobs, S. E., Ray, R. D., John, O. P., & Gross, J. J. (2012). Individual differences in reappraisal ability: Links to reappraisal frequency, well-being, and cognitive control. *Journal of Research in Personality, 46*(1), 2–7.

Minkel, J. D., McNealy, K., Gianaros, P. J., Drabant, E. M., Gross, J. J., Manuck, S. B., & Hariri, A. R. (2012). Sleep quality and neural circuit function supporting emotion regulation. *Biology of Mood & Anxiety Disorders, 2*(1), 22.

Morris, A. S., Silk, J. S., Steinberg, L., Myers, S. S., & Robinson, L. R. (2007). The role of the family context in the development of emotion regulation. *Social Development, 16*(2), 361–388.

Moser, J. S., Dougherty, A., Mattson, W. I., Katz, B., Moran, T. P., Guevarra, D., . . . Kross, E. (2017). Third-person self-talk facilitates emotion regulation without engaging cognitive control: Converging evidence from ERP and fMRI. *Scientific Reports, 7*(1), 4519.

Ochsner, K. N., & Gross, J. J. (2008). Cognitive emotion regulation: Insights from social cognitive and affective neuroscience. *Current Directions in Psychological Science, 17*(2), 153–158.

Parkinson, B., & Totterdell, P. (1999). Classifying affect-regulation strategies. *Cognition & Emotion, 13*(3), 277–303.

Pbert, L., Madison, J. M., Druker, S., Olendzki, N., Magner, R., Reed, G., . . . Carmody, J. (2012). Effect of mindfulness training on asthma quality of life and lung function: A randomized controlled trial. *Thorax, 67*(9), 769–776.

Petruzzello, S. J., Landers, D. M., Hatfield, B. D., Kubitz, K. A., & Salazar, W. (1991). A meta-analysis on the anxiety-reducing effects of acute and chronic exercise. *Sports Medicine, 11*(3), 143–182.

Porter, C. L. (2003). Coregulation in mother-infant dyads: Links to infants' cardiac vagal tone. *Psychological Reports, 92*(1), 307–319.

Shakespeare, W., & Hibbard, G. R. (1994). *Hamlet.* Oxford: Oxford University Press.

Spencer, S. J., Korosi, A., Layé, S., Shukitt-Hale, B., & Barrientos, R. M. (2017). Food for thought: How nutrition impacts cognition and emotion. *npj Science of Food, 1*(1), 7.

Steel, P. (2007). The nature of procrastination: A meta-analytic and theoretical review of quintessential self-regulatory failure. *Psychological Bulletin, 133*(1), 65–94.

Ströhle, A. (2009). Physical activity, exercise, depression and anxiety disorders. *Journal of Neural Transmission, 116*(6), 777–784.

Tsuno, N., Besset, A., & Ritchie, K. (2005). Sleep and depression. *Journal of Clinical Psychiatry, 66*(10), 1254–1269.

Umberson, D., & Karas Montez, J. (2010). Social relationships and health: A flashpoint for health policy. *Journal of Health and Social Behavior, 51*(Suppl), S54–S66.

Wehner, M. (2017, July 27). Talking to yourself isn't crazy, it's a stress relief. *New*

York Post. Retrieved from https://nypost.com/2017/07/27/talking-to-yourself-isnt
-crazy-its-stress-relief/

Wielgosz, J., Schuyler, B. S., Lutz, A., & Davidson, R. J. (2016). Long-term mindfulness training is associated with reliable differences in resting respiration rate. *Scientific Reports, 6,* 27533.

9. Emotions at Home

AVG Technologies. (2015, June 24). Kids competing with mobile phones for parents' attention [Web log message]. Retrieved from https://now.avg.com/digital-diaries
-kids-competing-with-mobile-phones-for-parents-attention

Baumeister, R. F., Bratslavsky, E., Finkenauer, C., & Vohs, K. D. (2001). Bad is stronger than good. *Review of General Psychology, 5*(4), 323–370. doi:10.1037//1089-2680.5.4.323

Bigelow, K. M., & Morris, E. K. (2001). John B. Watson's advice on child rearing: Some historical context. *Behavioral Development Bulletin, 10*(1), 26–30. http://dx.doi.org/10.1037/h0100479

Bowlby, J. (1988). *A Secure Base: Parent-Child Attachment and Healthy Human Development.* New York: Basic Books.

Boyce, T. W. (2019). *The Orchid and the Dandelion: Why Some Children Struggle and How All Can Thrive.* New York: Alfred A. Knopf.

Cacioppo, J. T., & Gardner, W. L. (1999). Emotion. *Annual Review of Psychology, 50*(1), 191–214. doi:10.1146/annurev.psych.50.1.191

Chaplin, T. M., & Aldao, A. (2013). Gender differences in emotion expression in children: A meta-analytic review. *Psychological Bulletin, 139*(4), 735–765. doi:10.1037/a0030737

DeClaire, J., & Gottman, J. (1997). *The Heart of Parenting: How to Raise an Emotionally Intelligent Child.* New York: Simon & Schuster.

Denham, S. A., Cook, M., & Zoller, D. (1992). "Baby looks *very* sad": Implications of conversations about feelings between mother and preschooler. *British Journal of Developmental Psychology, 10*(3), 301–315. doi.org/10.1111/j.2044-835X.1992.tb00579.x

Fogel, A. (1993). *Developing Through Relationships.* Chicago, IL: University of Chicago Press.

Hooven, C., Gottman, J. M., & Katz, L. F. (1995). Parental meta-emotion structure predicts family and child outcomes. *Cognition & Emotion, 9*(2–3), 229–264. doi.org/10.1080/02699939508409010

Johnson, D. J. (2017). Parents' perceptions of smartphone use and parenting practices. (Master's thesis). University of Nevada, Las Vegas. Available from Digital Scholarship@UNLV database. (No. 3141)

McDaniel, B. T., & Radesky, J. S. (2018). Technoference: Longitudinal associations between parent technology use, parenting stress, and child behavior problems. *Pediatric Research, 84*(2), 210–218. doi.org/10.1038/s41390-018-0052-6

Moore, S. D., Brody, L. R., & Dierberger, A. E. (2009). Mindfulness and experiential avoidance as predictors and outcomes of the narrative emotional disclosure task. *Journal of Clinical Psychology, 65*(9), 971–988. doi.org/10.1002/jclp.20600

Myruski, S., Gulyayeva, O., Birk, S., Pérez-Edgar, K., Buss, K. A., & Dennis-Tiwary, T. A. (2018). Digital disruption? Maternal mobile device use is related to infant social-emotional functioning. *Developmental Science, 21*(4), e12610. doi.org/10.1111/desc.12610

Ouellet-Morin, I., Odgers, C. L., Danese, A., Bowes, L., Shakoor, S., Papadopoulos, A. S., . . . Arseneault, L. (2011). Blunted cortisol responses to stress signal social and behavioral problems among maltreated/bullied 12-year-old children. *Biological Psychiatry, 70*(11), 1016–1023. doi.org/10.1016/j.biopsych.2011.06.017

Pew Research Center. (2018). *Teens, social media & technology 2018.* Retrieved from www.pewinternet.org/2018/05/31/teens-social-media-technology-2018/

Radesky, J. S., Kistin, C. J., Zuckerman, B., Nitzberg, K., Gross, J., Kaplan-Sanoff, M., . . . Silverstein, M. (2014). Patterns of mobile device use by caregivers and children during meals in fast food restaurants. *Pediatrics, 133*(4), e843–e849. Retrieved from https://pediatrics.aappublications.org/content/pediatrics/133/4/e843.full.pdf

Reed, J., Hirsh-Pasek, K., & Golinkoff, R. M. (2017). Learning on hold: Cell phones sidetrack parent-child interactions. *Developmental Psychology, 53*(8), 1428–1436. doi.org/10.1037/dev0000292

Rozin, P., & Royzman, E. B. (2001). Negativity bias, negativity dominance, and contagion. *Personality and Social Psychology Review, 5*(4), 296–320. doi.org/10.1207/S15327957PSPR0504_2

Steiner-Adair, C., & Barker, T. H. (2013). *The Big Disconnect: Protecting Childhood and Family Relationships in the Digital Age.* New York: Harper Business.

Stelter, R. L., & Halberstadt, A. G. (2011). The interplay between parental beliefs about children's emotions and parental stress impacts children's attachment security. *Infant and Child Development, 20*(3), 272–287. doi.org/10.1002/icd.693

Teicher, M. H., Samson, J. A., Sheu, Y. S., Polcari, A., & McGreenery, C. E. (2010). Hurtful words: Association of exposure to peer verbal abuse with elevated psychiatric symptom scores and corpus callosum abnormalities. *American Journal of Psychiatry, 167*(12), 1464–1471. doi.org/10.1176/appi.ajp.2010.10010030

Twenge, J. M., & Campbell, W. K. (2018). Associations between screen time and lower psychological well-being among children and adolescents: Evidence from

a population-based study. *Preventive Medicine Reports, 12,* 271–283. doi.org/10
.1016/j.pmedr.2018.10.003

U.S. Department of Education, National Center for Education Statistics. (2015). Student reports of bullying and cyber-bullying: Results from the 2013 School Crime Supplement to the National Crime Victimization Survey (NCES No. 2015–056). Retrieved from https://nces.ed.gov/pubs2015/2015056.pdf

Vaillancourt, T., Hymel, S., & McDougall, P. (2013). The biological underpinnings of peer victimization: Understanding why and how the effects of bullying can last a lifetime. *Theory into Practice, 52*(4), 241–248. doi.org/10.1080/00405841.2013 .829726

10. Emotions at School: From Preschool to College

Anxiety and Depression Association of America. Facts & statistics. Retrieved from https://adaa.org/about-adaa/press-room/facts-statistics

Aspen Institute National Commission on Social, Emotional, and Academic Development. (2019). From a nation at risk to a nation at hope. Retrieved from http://nationathope.org/wp-content/uploads/2018_aspen_final-report_full _webversion.pdf

Belfield, C., Bowden, A. B., Klapp, A., Levin, H., Shand, R., & Zander, S. (2015). The economic value of social and emotional learning. *Journal of Benefit-Cost Analysis, 6*(3), 508–544. doi.org/10.1017/bca.2015.55

Bell, C. C., & Jenkins, E. J. (1993). Community violence and children on Chicago's southside. *Psychiatry, 56*(1), 46–54. doi.org/10.1080/00332747.1993.11024620

Belsky, J., & de Haan, M. (2011). Annual research review: Parenting and children's brain development: The end of the beginning. *Journal of Child Psychology and Psychiatry, 52*(4), 409–428. doi.org/10.1111/j.1469-7610.2010.02281.x

Boyne, J. (2006). *The Boy in the Striped Pajamas.* Oxford: David Fickling Books.

Brackett, M. A., Elbertson, N. A., & Rivers, S. E. (2016). Applying theory to the development of approaches to SEL. In J. A. Durlak, C. E. Domitrovich, R. P. Weissberg, & T. P. Gullotta (Eds.), *Handbook of Social and Emotional Learning: Research and Practice* (pp. 20–32). New York: Guilford Press.

Brackett, M. A., Reyes, M. R., Rivers, S. E., Elbertson, N. A., & Salovey, P. (2011). Classroom emotional climate, teacher affiliation, and student conduct. *Journal of Classroom Interaction,* 27–36. Retrieved from www.jstor.org/stable/23870549

Brackett, M. A., Rivers, S. E., Reyes, M. R., & Salovey, P. (2012). Enhancing academic performance and social and emotional competence with the RULER feeling words curriculum. *Learning and Individual Differences, 22,* 218–224. doi.org /10.1016/j.lindif.2010.10.002

Bradley, C., Floman, J. L., Brackett, M. A., & Patti, J. (2019). Burnout and teacher well-being: The moderating role of perceived principal emotional intelligence. (Unpublished data.) Yale University, New Haven, CT.

Brooks, D. (2019, January 17). Students learn from people they love. *New York Times.* Retrieved from www.nytimes.com/2019/01/17/opinion/learning-emotion-education.html

Castillo, R., Fernández-Berrocal, P., & Brackett, M. A. (2013). Enhancing teacher effectiveness in Spain: A pilot study of the RULER approach to social and emotional learning. *Journal of Education and Training Studies, 1*(2), 263–272. doi.org/10.11114/jets.v1i2.203

Center for Collegiate Mental Health. (2016). *2015 annual report* (Publication No. STA 15-108). Retrieved from https://sites.psu.edu/ccmh/files/2017/10/2015_CCMH_Report_1-18-2015-yq3vik.pdf

Collaborative for Academic, Social, and Emotional Learning. (2015). Effective social and emotional learning programs. Retrieved from http://secondaryguide.casel.org/casel-secondary-guide.pdf

Divecha, D. & Brackett, M. A. (in press). Rethinking school-based bullying prevention through the lens of social and emotional learning: A bioecological perspective. *International Journal of Bullying Prevention.*

Durlak, J. A., Weissberg, R. P., Dymnicki, A. B., Taylor, R. D., & Schellinger, K. B. (2011). The impact of enhancing students' social and emotional learning: A meta-analysis of school-based universal interventions. *Child Development, 82*(1), 405–432. doi.org/10.1111/j.1467-8624.2010.01564.x

Gershoff, E. T., & Font, S. A. (2016). Corporal punishment in US public schools: Prevalence, disparities in use, and status in state and federal policy. *Social Policy Report, 30,* 1–37.

Gladden, R. M., Vivolo-Kantor, A. M., Hamburger, M. E., & Lumpkin, C. D. (2014). Bullying surveillance among youths: Uniform definitions for public health and recommended data elements, version 1.0. National Center for Injury Prevention and Control, Centers for Disease Control and Prevention, and U.S. Department of Education. Retrieved from www.cdc.gov/violenceprevention/pdf/bullying-definitions-final-a.pdf

Goleman, D. (1995). *Emotional Intelligence: Why It Can Matter More Than IQ.* New York: Bantam Books.

Greenberg, M. T., Brown, J. L., & Abenavoli, R. M. (2016, September). *Teacher stress and health: Effects on teachers, students, and schools.* Edna Bennett Pierce Prevention Research Center, Pennsylvania State University. Retrieved from www.rwjf.org/en/library/research/2016/07/teacher-stress-and-health.html

Holzapfel, B. (2018, January 20). Class of 2030: What do today's kindergartners need to be life-ready? [Web log message]. Retrieved from https://educationblog .microsoft.com/en-us/2018/01/class-of-2030-predicting-student-skills/

Immordino-Yang, M. H. (2015). *Emotions, Learning, and the Brain: Exploring the Educational Implications of Affective Neuroscience.* (Norton series on the social neuroscience of education). New York: W. W. Norton & Company.

Lipson, S. K., Lattie, E. G., & Eisenberg, D. (2018). Increased rates of mental health service utilization by US college students: 10-year population-level trends (2007–2017). *Psychiatric Services, 70*(1), 60–63. doi.org/10.1176/appi.ps.201800332

Loveless, T. (2017). 2017 Brown center report on American education: Race and school suspensions. Retrieved from www.brookings.edu/research/2017-brown -center-report-part-iii-race-and-school-suspensions/

McGraw-Hill Education. (2018). 2018 social and emotional learning report. Retrieved from www.mheducation.com/prek-12/explore/sel-survey.html

Microsoft Education. (2018). The class of 2030 and life-ready learning. Retrieved from https://education.minecraft.net/wp-content/uploads/13679_EDU_Thought _Leadership_Summary_revisions_5.10.18.pdf

Moeller, J., Ivcevic, Z., Brackett, M. A., & White, A. E. (2018). Mixed emotions: Network analyses of intra-individual co-occurrences within and across situations. *Emotion, 18*(8), 1106–1121. doi.org/10.1037/emo0000419

Murphey, D., Bandy, T., Schmitz, H., & Moore, K. (2013). Caring adults: Important for positive child well-being. *Child Trends.* Retrieved from www.childtrends.org /wp-content/uploads/2013/12/2013-54CaringAdults.pdf

Nathanson, L., Rivers, S. E., Flynn, L. M., & Brackett, M. A. (2016). Creating emotionally intelligent schools with RULER. *Emotion Review, 8*(4), 305–310. doi.org /10.1177/1754073916650495

New York State Education Department, New York City Department of Education. (2016). Memorandum of understanding. Retrieved from www.nysed.gov/common /nysed/files/DOE_MOU_FINAL.pdf

Parthenon-EY Education Practice, Ernst & Young LLP. (2016, September). Untapped potential: Engaging all Connecticut youth. Retrieved from http://cdn.ey.com /parthenon/pdf/perspectives/Parthenon-EY_Untapped-Potential_Dalio-Report _final_092016_web.pdf

Reyes, M. R., Brackett, M. A., Rivers, S. E., White, M., & Salovey, P. (2012). Classroom emotional climate, student engagement, and academic achievement. *Journal of Educational Psychology, 104*(3), 700–712. doi.org/10.1037/a0027268

Rivers, S. E., Brackett, M. A., Reyes, M. R., Elbertson, N. A., & Salovey, P. (2013). Improving the social and emotional climate of classrooms: A clustered randomized controlled trial testing the RULER Approach. *Prevention Science: The Official*

Journal of the Society for Prevention Research, 14, 77–87. doi.org/10.1007/s11121
-012-0305-2

Salovey, P., & Mayer, J. D. (1990). Emotional intelligence. *Imagination, Cognition and Personality, 9*(3), 185–211. doi.org/10.2190/DUGG-P24E-52WK-6CDG

Simmons, D. N., Brackett, M.A., & Adler, N. (2018, June). Applying an equity lens to social, emotional, and academic development. Edna Bennett Pierce Prevention Research Center, Pennsylvania State University. Retrieved from www.rwjf.org /en/library/research/2018/06/applying-an-equity-lens-to-social-emotional-and -academic-development.html

Sperduto, C., Kershaw, T., Brackett, M. A., & Monin, J. (in preparation). An app-based, emotional intelligence intervention for wellbeing in university students. Yale School of Medicine, Child Study Center, Yale University, New Haven, CT.

Taylor, R. D., Oberle, E., Durlak, J. A., & Weissberg, R. P. (2017). Promoting positive youth development through school-based social and emotional learning interventions: A meta-analysis of follow-up effects. *Child Development, 88*(4), 1156–1171. doi.org/10.1111/cdev.12864

White, A. E., Moeller, J., Ivcevic, Z., Brackett, M. A., & Stern, R. (2018). LGBTQ adolescents' positive and negative emotions and experiences in US high schools. *Sex Roles, 79*(9–10), 594–608. doi.org/10.1007/s11199-017-0885-1

11. Emotions at Work

Barsade, S. G. (2002). The ripple effect: Emotional contagion and its influence on group behavior. *Administrative Science Quarterly, 47*(4), 644–675.

Barsade, S. G., Brief, A. P., & Spataro, S. E. (2003). The affective revolution in organizational behavior: The emergence of a paradigm. *Organizational Behavior: The State of the Science, 2*, 3–52.

Barsade, S. G., & Gibson, D. E. (2007). Why does affect matter in organizations? *Academy of Management Perspectives, 21*(1), 36–59.

Barsade, S. G., & O'Neill, O. A. (2014). What's love got to do with it? A longitudinal study of the culture of companionate love and employee and client outcomes in a long-term care setting. *Administrative Science Quarterly, 59*(4), 551–598.

Caruso, D. R., & Salovey, P. (2004). *The Emotionally Intelligent Manager: How to Develop and Use the Four Key Emotional Skills of Leadership.* Hoboken, NJ: John Wiley & Sons.

Côté, S. (2014). Emotional intelligence in organizations. *Annual Review of Organizational Psychology and Organizational Behavior, 1*(1), 459–488.

Côté, S., Lopes, P. N., Salovey, P., & Miners, C. T. (2010). Emotional intelligence and leadership emergence in small groups. *Leadership Quarterly, 21*(3), 496–508.

David, S. (2016). *Emotional Agility.* New York: Penguin Group.

Grandey, A. A. (2003). When "the show must go on": Surface acting and deep acting as determinants of emotional exhaustion and peer-rated service delivery. *Academy of Management Journal, 46*(1), 86–96.

Harter, J. (2018, August 26). Employee engagement on the rise in the U.S. *Gallup News.* Retrieved from https://news.gallup.com/poll/241649/employee-engagement-rise .aspx

Hatfield, E., Cacioppo, J. T., & Rapson, R. L. (1993). Emotional contagion. *Current Directions in Psychological Science, 2*(3), 96–100.

Hennig-Thurau, T., Groth, M., Paul, M., & Gremler, D. D. (2006). Are all smiles created equal? How emotional contagion and emotional labor affect service relationships. *Journal of Marketing, 70*(3), 58–73.

Ivcevic, Z., Moeller, J., Menges, J., & Brackett, M. A. (under review). Supervisor emotionally intelligent behavior and employee creativity. *Journal of Creative Behavior.*

Knight, A. P., Menges, J. I., & Bruch, H. (2018). Organizational affective tone: A meso perspective on the origins and effects of consistent affect in organizations. *Academy of Management Journal, 61*(1), 191–219.

LaPalme, M. L., Rojas, F., Pertuzé, J. A., & Espinoza, P. Surface acting can be good . . . or bad: The influence of expressing inauthentic emotions on burnout, absenteeism, commitment, and patient complaints. (Manuscript submitted for publication).

Mayer, J. D., Roberts, R. D., & Barsade, S. G. (2008). Human abilities: Emotional intelligence. *Annual Review of Psychology, 59*, 507–536.

Menges, J. I. (2012). Organizational emotional intelligence: Theoretical foundations and practical implications. In C. E. J. Härtel, W. J. Zerbe, & N. M. Ashkanasy (Eds.), *Research on Emotions in Organizations* (vol. 8, pp. 355–373). Bingley, UK: Emerald.

Menges, J. I., & Bruch, H. (2009). Organizational emotional intelligence and performance: An empirical study. In C. E. J. Härtel, W. J. Zerbe, & N. M. Ashkanasy (Eds.), *Research on Emotions in Organizations* (vol. 5, pp. 181–209). Bingley, UK: Emerald.

Moeller, J., Ivcevic, Z., White, A. E., Menges, J. I., & Brackett, M. A. (2018). Highly engaged but burned out: Intra-individual profiles in the US workforce. *Career Development International, 23*(1), 86–105.

Rosete, D., & Ciarrochi, J. (2005). Emotional intelligence and its relationship to workplace performance outcomes of leadership effectiveness. *Leadership & Organization Development Journal, 26*(5), 388–399.

Schoenewolf, G. (1990). Emotional contagion: Behavioral induction in individuals and groups. *Modern Psychoanalysis, 15*(1), 49–61.

Seppälä, E. & Moeller, J. (2018, January 2). 1 in 5 employees is highly engaged and at risk of burnout. *Harvard Business Review*. Retrieved from https://hbr.org/2018/02/1-in-5-highly-engaged-employees-is-at-risk-of-burnout

Taylor, C., Ivcevic, Z., Moeller, J., & Brackett, M. A. (under review). Gender and creativity at work. *Creativity and Innovation Management*.

Acknowledgments

I have immense gratitude for the countless people and organizations that have contributed to my personal and professional growth and to the contents in this book.

I would first like to thank my wonderful agent, Richard Pine, and the team at Inkwell Management, especially Eliza Rothstein, William Callahan, and Lyndsey Blessing, for all their guidance and care through every stage of the publishing process. I also thank Amy Hertz who, early on, was instrumental in helping me shape the structure of this book. I'm grateful for Bill Tonelli, who supported me throughout the writing of this book, and especially for helping me make my own and others' academic research accessible for a broad audience.

I cannot say thank you enough times to the dedicated and talented people at Celadon Books, my publisher, who have been far more encouraging than I had imagined possible, including: Jamie Raab, my editor and publisher, and the entire team: Deb Futter, Rachel Chou, Ryan Doherty, Anne Twomey, Christie Mykityshyn, Heather Graham, Jaime Noven, Randi Kramer, Alexis Neuville, Cecily Van Buren-Freedman, and Clay Smith. Their suggestions, support, and especially all of their excitement about my ideas have made my dream of writing this book a reality.

Over the last twenty-five years, I have had the unique privilege of working with talented educators in thousands of schools across the United States and in other countries. I learned something from each person and school with whom I've interacted, particularly those schools and districts that participated in my research or shared their stories with me. I send a special shout-out to Valley Stream District 24 on Long Island and Ed Fale and Bruce Alster, who partnered with our team to do RULER's very first study over fifteen years ago. A second shout-out goes to the Roman Catholic Diocese of Brooklyn and Queens, and especially their former district administrator, Michael Pizzingrillo, who was instrumental in our first randomized controlled trial of RULER. I extend deep gratitude to the NYC Department of Education with special thank-yous to Dolores Esposito, Carmen Fariña, LeShawn Robinson, Richard Carranza, Brooke Jackson, Dawn DeCosta, and David Adams. I am eternally grateful to Bonnie Brown, who brought RULER into NYC's special education District 75, helping us reach thousands of children with emotional challenges and those on the autism spectrum.

Other schools to whom I'm indebted include our early adopters and partners: New Line Learning, especially Chris Gerry and Clare Collins; Girton Grammar, especially Paul Flanagan, Les Evans, and Matthew Maruff; Brewster Academy, especially Mike Cooper and Allie Cooper; the Shipley School, especially Steven Piltch; Horace Mann, especially Deena Neuwirth and Tom Kelly; Prospect Sierra, especially Katherine Dinh and Heather Rogers; Seattle Public Schools, especially Helen Walsh and Bryan Manzo; Highline Public Schools, especially Susan Enfield, Laurie Morrison, and Kimberly Kinzer; Fairfax County Public Schools, especially MaryAnn Panarelli, Dede Bailor, and Jeanne Veraska; Aidan Montessori, especially Kathy Minardi; Bridgeport Public Schools, especially Fran Rabinowitz for her vision; Technológico de Monterrey, especially Paulino Bernot Silis and Rafael

Abrego Hinojosa; Academy District 20 in Colorado Springs, especially Susan Field, Maureen Lang, and Clark Maxon; the King David School, especially David Opat; Hamden Public Schools, especially Valerie Larose; Joel Barlow High School, and in particular, Gina-Marie Pin and Chris Poulos; and Coquitlam District No. 43, especially Tamara Banks.

I also want to thank key partners who have helped us scale RULER across the United States, including the Willows Community School, notably Lisa Rosenstein, Susan Sleeper, and Christina Kim, and Putnam North West BOCES in New York, especially Renee Gargano and Joan Thompson. In our journey to make Connecticut the first emotionally intelligent state, I want to acknowledge our biggest champions: Dianna Wentzel, commissioner of education; Fran Rabinowitz, executive director of the Connecticut Association of Public School Superintendents; Bob Rader, executive director of the Connecticut Association of Boards of Education; and Steven Hernandez, executive director of the Connecticut Commission on Women, Children, and Seniors. We wouldn't have reached a fraction of the children and educators in Connecticut and New York without their passion and dedication.

Our center's research and approach to SEL, RULER, was made possible with the support from these generous organizations: Anthony and Jeanne Pritzker Family Foundation, Arnow Family Foundation, Chan Zuckerberg Initiative (Brooke Stafford-Brizard, Gaby López, and Priscilla Chan), Corbett Family Foundation, Dalio Foundation (Barbara Dalio, Andrew Ferguson, Kevin Ashley), Dancing Tides Foundation, Einhorn Family Charitable Trust (Jennifer Hoos Rothberg and Itai Dinour), Faas Foundation (Andy Faas and Patrick Mundt), Facebook (Arturo Bejar and Jamie Lockwood), La Fundacíon Botín (Íñigo Sáenz and Fátima Sánchez), Graustein Memorial Fund, Greater Houston Community Foundation, Hartford Foundation (Richard Sussman), Hauptman Family Foundation, Institute for Education Science, Institute for Social Policy Studies at Yale, Lurie Family Foundation, The Meeting House (Paula Resnick), Novo Foundation (Jennifer Buffet), Oxman Family Foundation, Partners of '63 (Charley Ellis and

Jim Schattinger), Phillipe Costeletos Family, Pure Edge (Chi Kim), Robert Wood Johnson (Jennifer Ng'andu and Tracy Costigan), Seedlings Foundation (Karen Pritzker and Kathy Higgins), Simms/Mann Foundation, Susan Crowne Exchange (Susan Crowne and Haviland Rummel), Tauck Family Foundation (Mirellise Vazquez), Wallace Foundation (Gigi Antoni and Katherine Lewandoski), Wend Ventures (Nora Flood), William T. Grant Foundation, World Wrestling Entertainment, Inc., and Yale China Fund for Emotional Intelligence (Neil Shen and Leon Meng).

I also extend my deepest appreciation to many others who have contributed to this book, including Daniel Goleman, who helped me find my mentors, Peter Salovey and Jack Mayer; Richard and Susan Reiner; Mark Sparvell (Microsoft); Denise Daniels (Moodsters); Barbara Winston and Stephanie Winston Wolkoff (UN Women for Peace Association); Jeannie Francolini (Flawless Foundation); Ginny Deering and Bridget Durkan Laird (Wings); Bill Jackson (Great Schools); Crystal Brown (Boys and Girls Clubs of America); Leslie Udwin (Think Equal); Roger Weissberg, Karen Niemi, and Tim Shriver (CASEL); Wendy Baron and Ellen Moir (New Teacher Center); Christopher Rim (Command Education); and HopeLab, especially Fred Dillan, Brian Rodriquez, and Shane Brentham for their support in building and maintaining our Mood Meter App.

I want to thank those who shared their time and intellect in providing feedback to this manuscript: Dacher Keltner, Deb and Hugh Jackman, Diane Archer, Harriet Seittler, James Gross, Janet Patti, Jeff Clifford, Jochen Menges, Karen Niemi, Kathy Higgins, Jamie Lockwood, Roger Weissberg, Scott Levy, Sigal Barsade, Tara Westover, Tim Shriver, Jennifer Allen, and Zorana Ivcevic.

My research and thinking throughout the years have been influenced by countless other researchers and practitioners, including: Angela Duckworth, Carol Dweck, Dan Siegel, Erica Frydenberg, Kim Schonert-Reichl, Lisa Feldman Barrett, Mark Greenberg, Maurice Elias, Miriam Miller, Pam Cantor, Patricia Lester, Richard Durlak, Roger Weissberg,

Stephanie Jones, Tim Shriver, Shauna Tominey, and Sharon Shapses. I also thank my mentors and friends from the martial arts, who no doubt contributed to my views. And, I send special thank-yous to Doc Krawiec, Bob Bross, Mike Wollmershauser, Grand Master Im Hyun Soo, and my friend and martial arts partner for over thirty years, Michael D'Aloia. For the last fifteen years, I've also had two incredible yoga teachers I want to thank for their contributions to my mindset: Peg Olivera and Lori Bonazzoli. And, I owe my physical and mental health to Damian Paglia's relentless efforts.

I extend my gratitude to my partners at Oji Life Lab, including Matt Kursh, Andrea Hoban, and Camilla Mize, all of whom gave great feedback on this manuscript; to Diana Divecha and Robin Stern, who were with me every step of the way, reading multiple versions of each chapter; and James Floman, Nikki Elbertson, and Kathryn Lee, whose extensive feedback and editorial guidance enhanced this book. I want to give a special thank-you to Christina Bradley, who helped me gather the resources for this book and worked with me on the bibliography.

My colleagues, students, and research team over the last twenty years have made my career a complete joy. This work benefited enormously from Jack Mayer, Peter Salovey, and David Caruso. Each of these individuals has been an incredible mentor and colleague. Robin Stern and Janet Patti also have a special place in my heart for supporting my journey. Charley Ellis has been a tremendous mentor to me and I'm forever grateful for his guidance and support.

At Yale, I have many people to thank, including Linda Mayes, Kim Goff Crews, James Comer, Edward Zigler, and Heidi Brooks. At the Yale Center for Emotional Intelligence, we have been blessed with hundreds of talented individuals. I am especially grateful to Susan Rivers and Robin Stern, who were my co-founders. Susan and I conducted most of the original research on RULER while Robin and I worked together with David Caruso on the original RULER training materials. Their wisdom is spread throughout this book. Our current senior leadership team, which includes Scott Levy, Dena Simmons, and Robin Stern, provided tremendous support during the writing of this book. And Michelle Lugo, my executive assistant and daily partner, provided her unconditional support every step of the way in writing this book. Michelle—I would not have been able to write this book without you!

I also have tremendous gratitude for the dedication and creativity of our center directors, Danica Kelly, Christina Cipriano, Andrés Richner, Nikki Elbertson, and James Hagen, and our project directors and lead researchers, including Craig Bailey, Jessica Hoffmann, Zorana Ivcevic, James Floman, Jennifer Allen, Kathryn Lee, Charlene Voyce, and Emma Seppälä. All of these talented people lead teams of program and research managers, all of whom have contributed to my thinking—and have made our center what it is today. I also want to acknowledge Laura Artusio and Ruth Gualdo Castillo, who direct our work in Italy and Spain, respectively.

Above all, I thank my family for their love and encouragement. My parents, William and Diane Brackett; my brother, Steven Nadler, and my sister-in-law, Leticia Fraga Nadler, and their children, Benjamin and Sofia; my brother, David Nadler; my cousin Ellyn Solis and her daughter, Esme; and my cousins Richard and Lisa Maurer and their children, Jared, Jacob, and Megan. I also hold enormous gratitude for my mother-in-law, Irene; my aunt, Sandra Price; and Jane Brackett. Words cannot express my deepest gratitude to my partner of twenty-five years and husband of nine years, Horacio Marquínez. His love and commitment to me and my work goes beyond any expectation of a life partner.

This book is about personal growth and transformation through unlocking the wisdom of emotions. Writing it has given me greater insight into my own emotional life and inspired me to further develop my own emotion skills, and I hope it has done the same for you. So, last but not least, I thank you, the reader, for allowing me and this book to guide you through that journey.